Dropout Prevention Tools

Franklin P. Schargel

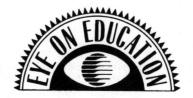

EYE ON EDUCATION
6 DEPOT WAY WEST, SUITE 106
LARCHMONT, NY 10538
(914) 833–0551
(914) 833–0761 fax
www.eyeoneducation.com

Library of Congress Cataloging-in-Publication Data

Dropout prevention tools / edited by Franklin P. Schargel.
      p. cm.
   ISBN 1-930556-52-7
   1. Dropouts--United States--Prevention. 2. School improvement programs--United States. 3. Educational change--United States. I. Schargel, Franklin P.

LC143.D76 2003
371.2'913--dc21

                                                     2002192867

10 9 8 7 6 5 4 3 2

Editorial and production services provided by
Richard H. Adin Freelance Editorial Services
52 Oakwood Blvd., Poughkeepsie, NY 12603-4112
(845-471-3566)

Also available from Eye On Education

Strategies to Help Solve Our School Dropout Problem
Franklin P. Schargel and Jay Smink

Achievement Now!
How to Assure No Child is Left Behind
Dr. Donald J. Fielder

Student Transitions from Middle to High School:
Improving Achievement and Creating a Safer Environment
J. Allen Queen

The Directory of Programs for Students at Risk
Thomas Williams

Constructivist Strategies:
Meeting Standards and Engaging Adolescent Minds
Foote, Vermette, and Battaglia

Beyond Vocational Education:
Career Majors, Tech Prep, Schools Within Schools,
Magnet Schools, and Academies
David Pucel

Dealing with Difficult Parents
(And with Parents in Difficult Situations)
Whitaker and Fiore

101 "Answers" for New Teachers and Their Mentors:
Effective Teaching Tips for Daily Classroom Use
Annette Breaux

Motivating and Inspiring Teachers:
The Educational Leader's Guide for Building Staff Morale
Todd Whitaker, Beth Whitaker, and Dale Lumpa

Performance Assessment and Standards-Based Curricula:
The Achievement Cycle
Allan Glatthorn, et al.

Performance Standards and Authentic Learning
Allan Glatthorn

DEDICATION

To the Schargels

Sandy, my life companion

and my children, David, Howie, and Pegi

Foreword

The initial book, *Strategies to Help Solve Our School Dropout Problem*, written by Franklin Schargel and me, was based on more than a decade of research and experiences by the National Dropout Prevention Center at Clemson University while working with schools and communities across the nation. The 15 strategies we identified reflected successful practices and interventions from the past decade. These same 15 strategies will likely remain a viable part of any school improvement plan developed by school and community leaders in the foreseeable future.

We were extremely gratified to receive so much interest in the initial book that it seemed natural to build on the 15 most effective strategies to solve the school dropout problem. Therefore, I encouraged Franklin to pursue the development of this second book, which builds on the base of the 15 strategies by offering the "best practices" developed and implemented in many successful schools and communities across the nation. Franklin has also included numerous program guidelines and recommendations from local, state, and federal agencies that carry responsibility for improving academic achievement and increasing the high school graduation rate.

This new book, *Dropout Prevention Tools*, offers readers a solid set of program recommendations and practical applications in each of the 15 strategies. These best practices represent just a small portion of the many successful policies and practices uncovered from around the nation; however, they offer school planners an excellent starting point and should be modified to fit the local culture and then implemented in schools and communities to complement and enhance other programs already underway.

As we stated in our earlier book, any of these best practices standing alone will have a positive impact on students, teachers, schools, and families. For the exceptional results, however, all of these practices should first be thoroughly studied to determine how they align with local program objectives and other current programs. The next step would be to assemble a combination of these practices to be fully integrated into the local school program and within the culture of the community. In summary, these practices—along with this suggested planning strategy—should provide local school and community leaders with the best results in student achievement and increased graduation rates. Good luck!

Jay Smink, Executive Director
National Dropout Prevention Center
Clemson University, Clemson, South Carolina

Acknowledgements

The creation of this book, more than most, depended on the expertise and knowledge of others. The contributions of many individuals and organizations have made this book possible. Their beneficence and willingness to share their knowledge about effective programs and interventions, as well as their desire to help others succeed, is a tribute to them. You will find their names, their schools or programs (including a short description), and their contact information at the end of the book.

I must thank a number of individuals who graciously shared their expertise with me. It is particularly because of the individuals named here and below that I was able to write this book: Jim Lockhart III and Judy Craig, United States Department of Education; Jennifer Yahn, New Mexico Department of Education; and Dr. John Humins and Carmine DeBetta, New York City Board of Education.

Early stages of this manuscript were reviewed by Linda E. Young, Karen Ann Goeller, Steven Kimberling, and Christopher Chalker.

I also give special thanks to Dr. Jay Smink, Executive Director of the National Dropout Prevention Center based at Clemson University, and his associates: Marty Duckenfield, Patricia Cloud Duttweiler, John Peters, Mary Reimer, Dr. Sam Drew, Dr. Terry Cash, Susie Turbeville, Dr. Ted Wesley, and Linda Shirley.

And a sincere thank you to Robert Sickles, my publisher, for is support, encouragement, and vision and his willingness to take a risk on this project.

Meet
Franklin P. Schargel

Franklin P. Schargel, a native of Brooklyn, New York, who now resides in Albuquerque, New Mexico, is a graduate of the University of the City of New York (City University). Mr. Schargel holds two master's degrees. His career spans 33 years of classroom teaching, 8 years as an assistant principal, and he taught a course in Dowling College's MBA program.

Mr. Schargel served on the Guidelines Development Committee for the Malcolm Baldrige National Quality Award in Education and was an examiner for the Baldrige Award. He also served as a judge for both the Secretary of the Air Force Quality Award and the USA Today/RIT Quality Cup. He currently serves as chair of the American Society of Quality's Education Division.

Mr. Schargel is the author of *Transforming Education Through Total Quality Management: A Practitioner's Guide*, as well as more than 50 articles published in leading educational journals and business magazines. *Dropout Prevention Tools* is a companion piece to *Strategies to Help Solve Our School Dropout Problem*, which was cowritten by Mr. Schargel and Dr. Jay Smink, Executive Director of the National Dropout Prevention Center at Clemson University. Mr. Schargel has a regular monthly Internet column at www.guidance channel.com as well as quarterly column in "Quality Education."

Mr. Schargel's success in dramatically enhancing the learning process at George Westinghouse High School in New York—by expanding parental involvement, increasing postsecondary school attendance, and significantly lowering the student dropout rate— has been documented in 25 books, 55 newspaper and magazine articles, and 5 internationally released videos.

As president of his training firm, The Schargel Consulting Group, Mr. Schargel has presented countless workshops for educational, community, and business groups throughout the United States, Europe, Canada, and Latin America. His workshops are for administrators, teachers, students, parents, business leaders, policymakers, and anyone else interested in building world-class schools. The workshops cover a wide variety of topics, including dealing with at-risk school populations, increasing the graduation rate for all students, consensus building, curriculum innovation, educational leadership, staff empowerment, interactive learning, learner-directed learning, the Malcolm Baldrige National Quality Award in Education, organizational change, parental involvement, problem solving, school-to-work programs, strategic planning, student evaluation and data analysis, teamwork, technological preparation, and total quality education. His workshops are tailored to the individual client's needs and expected outcomes. For additional information: He can be reached at Franklin@Schargel.com

Introduction

This book serves as a companion to *Strategies to Help Solve Our School Dropout Problem*. The strategies book, coauthored with Dr. Jay Smink, Executive Director of the National Dropout Prevention Center at Clemson University, supplied the "what-to-do." This book supplies the "how-to-do" it.

This toolkit provides "best practices" material that has been used successfully by schools, school districts, and a variety of state and local programs to help address the at-risk student population. The strategies book provides the foundation on which this toolkit rests. The tools in this book fit into the framework of the strategies. Whereas the strategies book addresses the macropicture, *Dropout Prevention Tools* focuses on the micropicture.

This book can be a most effective resource for those interested in establishing schools or programs to deal with at-risk students; for those currently involved in schools or programs; and for those who would like to improve what has already been done.

I have collected information from the United States Department of Education, state Departments of Education, colleagues, people I have met while presenting or attending workshops, schools and programs that have been identified as successfully recovering dropout students, and others that have prevented students from becoming potential dropouts. In addition, a number of my friends in the educational community have shared their successful practices.

Why Is There a Need For a Toolkit?

Educators want and need a set of reliable practices that will enable them to take advantage of what others have learned and to avoid the pitfalls others faced and conquered. The tools, rubrics, guiding ideas, and resources in this book illustrate how to apply the 15 strategies.

How to Read this Book

Like you, this book is unique, so there is no right way or wrong way to read it. It has been designed for easy use. You may want to start at the first page and go all the way through, or you might see a tool that intrigues you and will start there. Feel free to make the book your own, because it is. Mark up the book; highlight the "good parts." We have tried to make this book user-friendly in the following ways:

- ◆ CD-ROM

  This book comes with a CD-ROM from which all the tools can be accessed using Adobe Acrobat Reader®. Selected worksheets and forms are also available in Microsoft Word®. See page xiii for details.

- ◆ Modules

  This book is divided into 15 modules, 1 for each of the 15 strategies identified in the strategies book. Each module contains tools, graphs, charts, and rubrics pertaining to that particular strategy.

- ◆ Shaded Steps

  On the right-hand side of each tool, you will find shaded steps. These icons clarify the grade levels for which the tools are most appropriate. The grade levels are as follows:

Pre-school & Elementary

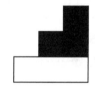
Elementary School

Middle & High School

All Grade Levels

- ◆ Icons

  In the strategies book, the strategies were separated from one another. Similarly, the activities in this manual are presented individually so the reader can investigate the different types of activities available. In reality, however, activities are rarely conducted independently. Highly effective schools and programs combine a number of strategies to render maximum impact on the dropout problem. For example, many strategies apply to more than one section of the book. At the top of the page is an icon indicating which strategy, or strategies, is applied by that particular technique. An icons key may be found on page .

- ◆ Indices

  Two indices break the activities into educational grade level (such as preschool, elementary, middle or junior high, and high school) and strategy.

Will the Exercises Work for Me?

All of the tools in this book have been field-tested. We know that these tools and techniques have worked and have produced positive results. However, each school has its own culture. The tools must be customized for your community. (Simply using them without adapting them to your culture will render their effectiveness suboptimal.) No one knows better than you what will work in your locale. I suggest that you try the tool the way it appears, then ask the people who have been involved in deployment of the tool how they would improve the tool or its deployment.

After you have tried the tool, ask yourself the following questions:

- ◆ What about this tool worked?
- ◆ What made it work?
- ◆ What needs to be improved or modified?
- ◆ How do we make those modifications?
- ◆ What do we have to measure to know that we have made the right improvements?

A Work in Progress

What you hold in your hands is a work in progress. It will surely need to be modified, expanded, and corrected. I would like to know what you did with the tools. What worked? What modifications made the tools work better? Do you have any tools or techniques that proved successful with at-risk students? If so, why not send them to me so we can include them in the next book of tools?

If would like to join me in this effort to supply our colleagues, America's children, their parents, and the business community in this crucial effort to end the phenomenon of school dropout, fill out the forms below. Please use one set of papers for each technique you submit. Please attach one permission slip for each separate technique. Do not send any material copyrighted by others. If you send *your* copyrighted material, please indicate so on the attached form.

If you wish to contact me, feel free to write me at franklin@schargel.com. To find out about the other work I am doing, see my Web site at www.schargel.com.

Franklin P. Schargel
Albuquerque, New Mexico

The CD—What's On It & How to Use It!

The CD accompanying this book has three directories:

(1) *E-book,* which includes a complete copy of the print version of this book in PDF format

(2) *Install Acrobat Reader,* which includes a free copy of the current version of Adobe Acrobat Reader® that you can install on your computer to access the PDF version of this book

(3) *Interactive Forms,* which contains electronic versions of some of the forms found in this book, enabling you to fill them out, customize them, and save and print them using Microsoft Word®

The E-book Directory

The entire book is available in electronic form in this directory and can be read on your computer screen as an e-book by using Adobe Acrobat Reader®.

You can search the e-book by clicking on an entry in the table of contents or the indexes. To print specific pages from the e-book version, choose **Print** on the **File Menu** and follow the instructions.

The Install Acrobat Reader Directory

If Adobe Acrobat Reader® is not already on your computer, a free copy of the current version is available on this CD-ROM and can be installed on your computer.

The Interactive Forms Directory

Many of the worksheets and forms showcased in *Dropout Prevention Tools* are interactive. These particular tools are available in Microsoft Word® format in this directory. You can fill them out electronically, save the completed forms as new, unique Word files, and print them.

Complete the form by typing in the blanks provided and/or by clicking on the checkboxes. Use the **Tab** key to move from field to field. When you are finished, save the file with a unique name by using the **Save As** function.

Worksheets and forms are "protected," that is, the instructions on the form and its structure are locked and cannot be changed unless you choose to do so. If you want to make modifications to the language on the form (such as inserting the name of your school or district, or otherwise customizing the language on the form) follow these directions:

(1) Choose **Unprotect Document** from the **Tools** menu.

(2) Type in the password "Modify" (it must be typed exactly as shown here; it is case sensitive) and click the OK button. The form will unlock and become a regular Word document.

(3) Save the file with a new name using the **Save As** function.

While a document is unprotected, form functionality is unavailable. To re-enable form functions, choose **Protect Document** from the **Tools** menu. Note that re-enabling a form will remove any data that you previously inserted into the form fields.

The interactive forms available on this CD are listed here; the files are named by their book page number:

- After-School Experiences
  Page 69.doc   Identifying staff training needs and resources
- Alternative Schooling
  Page 45.doc   Aligning Alternative Education Programs with Standards
  Page 52.doc   Monitoring Academic Performance
  Page 56.doc   Monitoring Student Behavior Using a Checklist
  Page 60.doc   Entering Middle and High School Student Self Assessment
- Diverse Learning Styles
  Page 98.doc   Occupation and Intelligences Chart
- Individualized Instruction
  Page 114.doc   Individual Learning Plan
- Professional Development
  Page 86.doc   Measuring the Success of Teaming Strategies
  Page 89.doc   Student Performance Self Evaluation Form
- Safe Schools
  Page 172.doc   In-School Suspension Letter to Parents
- Service Learning
  Page 39.doc   Learning Tracking Sheet
- Systemic Reform
  Page 143.doc   Measuring Your Organization's Progress

Permission and Help

Permission is granted to reproduce these forms for educational purposes providing the notice at the bottom of each page appears. This material may not be sold or repackaged without the written permission of the copyright holder and the publisher.

If you have any difficulty with the forms, accessing the e-book, or with installing Adobe Acrobat Reader®, please consult with your technology coordinator or network administrator. Eye On Education does not provide technical support.

Key to Tool Icons

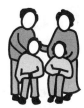

Family
Involvement

Early Childhood
Education

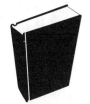

Reading/Writing
Programs

Mentoring
and Tutoring

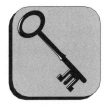

Service
Learning

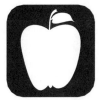

Alternative
Schooling

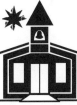

After School
Experiences

Professional
Development

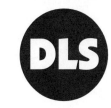

Diverse Learning Styles/
Multiple Intelligences

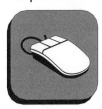

Instructional
Technology

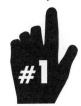

Individualized
Instruction

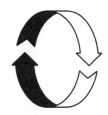

Systemic Renewal

Community
Collaboration

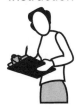

Career Education and
Workforce Readiness

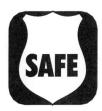

Safe Schools

What's Working in Your School or District?

As we make plans for the next volume of **Dropout Prevention Tools**, we invite you to send us your material so we can consider disseminating it.
For more details, please contact:

Franklin P. Schargel
10202 Jarash Place, NE
Albuquerque, NM 87122
Fax (505) 823-2339
franklin@schargel.com

Table of Contents

The 15 Effective Strategies Explained

Early Interventions

Family Involvement

Research consistently finds that family involvement has a direct, positive effect on children's achievement and is the most accurate predictor of a student's success in school.

Early Childhood Education

Interventions that take place between birth and three years demonstrate that providing a child with educational enrichment can modify IQ. The most effective way to decrease the number of children who will ultimately drop out is to provide the best possible classroom instruction from the beginning of the school experience.

Reading and Writing Programs

Early interventions to help low-achieving students recognize that focusing on reading and writing skills are the foundation for effective learning in all subjects.

The Basic Core Strategies

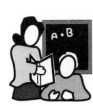

Mentoring and Tutoring

Mentoring is a one-to-one caring, supportive relationship between a mentor and a mentee that is based on trust. Tutoring, also a one-to-one activity, focuses on academics and is an effective way to address specific needs such as reading, writing, or math competencies.

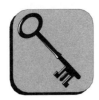

Service Learning

Service learning connects meaningful community service experiences with academic learning. This method for teaching and learning promotes personal and social growth, career development, and civic responsibility and can be a powerful vehicle for effective school reform at all grade levels.

Alternative Schooling
Alternative schooling provides potential dropouts with a variety of options that can lead to graduation, with programs paying special attention to the student's individual social needs and the academic requirements for a high school diploma.

After School Experiences
Many schools provide after-school and summer enhancement programs that eliminate information loss and inspire interest in a variety of areas. Such experiences are especially important for students at risk of school failure.

Making the Most of Instruction

No sustained and comprehensive effort to keep students in school can afford to ignore what happens in the classroom. Strategies that produce better teachers—by expanding teaching methods to accommodate a range of learning styles, taking advantage of today's cornucopia of technological resources, and meeting the individual needs of each student—yield substantial benefits.

Professional Development
Teachers who work with youth at high risk for academic failure need to feel supported and need to have an avenue by which they may continue to develop skills and techniques and learn innovative teaching strategies.

Diverse Learning Styles and Multiple Intelligences
When educators show students that there are different ways to learn, students find new and creative ways to solve problems, achieve success, and become lifelong learners.

Instructional Technologies
Technology offers some of the best opportunities for delivering instruction that engages students in authentic learning, addresses multiple intelligences, and adapts to students' learning styles.

Individualized Instruction
A customized individual learning program for each student allows teachers to be flexible with the instructional program and extracurricular activities.

Making the Most of the Wider Community

Students who come to school bring traces from a wider community; when students leave school, either before or after graduation, they return to that community. It is impossible to isolate "school" within the walls of the school building. Effective efforts to keep students in school take advantage of these links with the wider community.

Systemic Renewal

Systemic renewal calls for a continuing process of evaluating goals and objectives related to school policies, practices, and organizational structures as they impact a diverse group of learners.

Community Collaboration

When all groups in a community provide collective support to the school, a strong infrastructure sustains a caring environment in which youth can thrive and achieve.

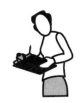

Career Education and Workforce Readiness

A quality guidance program is essential for all students. School- to-work programs recognize that youth need specific skills to prepare them for the larger demands of today's workplace.

Safe Schools

A comprehensive violence prevention plan, including conflict resolution, must deal with potential violence as well as crisis management. Violence prevention means providing daily experiences at all grade levels that enhance positive social attitudes and effective interpersonal skills in all students.

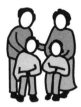

Family Involvement

Research consistently finds that family involvement has a direct, positive effect on children's achievement and is the most accurate predictor of a student's success in school. Tools in this module include:

"**How Parents Can Help Their Children Be Ready to Read,**" adapted from "A Guide For Reading: How Parents Can Help Their Children Be Ready to Read and Ready to Learn," White House Initiative on Educational Excellence for Hispanic Americans.

"**How Parents Can Help Their Young Children (Ages 2 to 5 Years) Learn Math,**" information taken from the United States Department of Education booklet, "Early Childhood: Where Learning Begins. Mathematics."

"**How Parents Can Help Their Children Avoid Alcohol and Drugs,**" adapted from "Growing Up Drug-Free: A Parent's Guide to Prevention," United States Department of Education, Office of Elementary and Secondary Education, Safe and Drug-Free Schools Program, published 1988.

"**What Parents Can Do if They Think Their Child May Be Taking Drugs,**" adapted from "Growing Up Drug-Free: A Parent's Guide to Prevention," United States Department of Education, Office of Elementary and Secondary Education, Safe and Drug-Free Schools Program, published 1988.

"**How to Prepare a Checklist for a Meeting with Parents and Guardians,**" developed by Steve Berta, Manager of Student Services and Guidance at San Jose Unified School District; Howard Blonsky, San Francisco Unified School District Trainer; Vicki Butler, Coordinator/Principal for Special Schools at the Riverside County Office of Education; Bill Deeb, Director of Research and Evaluation at Alisal Union School District; Marco Orlando, consultant with the California Department of Education; and Andy Stetkevich, Staff Development Specialist for the Riverside Unified School District. Used with the permission of Howard Blonsky.

How Parents Can Help
Their Children Be Ready to Read

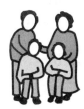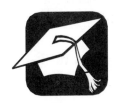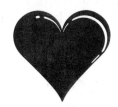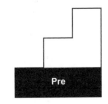

Parents are the first and, initially, the most important teachers. United States Department of Education data indicate that 91% of a child's growth period (age 5 to 18 years) is spent outside the school and classrooms. It is therefore essential to recruit parents to aid in the learning process.

- **Talk to your infant and toddler to help him learn to speak and understand the meaning of words.**

  Point to objects that are nearby, and describe them as you play and perform daily activities together. Sharing a large vocabulary gives your child a great start when he enters school.

- **Start reading to your baby every day starting at six months of age.**

  Reading and playing with books is a wonderful way to spend special time with her. Hearing words over and over helps her become familiar with them. Reading to your baby is one of the best ways to help her learn.

- **Use sounds, songs, gestures, and words that rhyme to help your baby learn about language and its main uses.**

  Babies need to hear language from a human being. To a baby, television is just noise.

- **Point out the printed words in your home and other places you take your child, such as the grocery store.**

  Spend as much time listening to your child as you do talking to him.

- **Take children's books and writing materials with you whenever you leave home.**

  Doing so gives your child fun activities to entertain and occupy her while traveling to the doctor's office and other appointments.

- **Create a quiet, special place in your home for your child to read, write, and draw.**

  Keep books and other reading materials where your child can easily reach them.

♦ **Limit the amount and type of television shows you and your child watch.**

Better yet, turn off the television, and spend more time cuddling and reading books with your child. The time and attention you give your child provides many benefits beyond helping him become ready to succeed in school.

♦ **Reach out to libraries and community and faith-based organizations. These organizations can do the following:**

- help you find age-appropriate books to use at home with your child;

- show you creative ways to use books with your child and other tips to help her learn; and

- provide year-round reading and educational activities for your child.

How Parents Can Help Their Young Children (Ages 2 to 5 Years) Learn Math

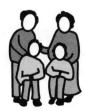  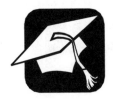 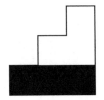

Children need help with reading and mathematics as they are growing up. The United States Department of Education has developed strategies to help parents assist their young children with mathematics.

- Help your child find patterns in designs and pictures.
- Sort objects by looking for similarities in color, shape, or size.
- Sort objects by looking for differences, such as determining which object is bigger or smaller.
- Use traffic signs to help children learn different shapes. For example, a yield sign is shaped like a triangle, and a stop sign is shaped like an octagon.
- Sing songs that rhyme, repeat, or have numbers in them. Examples include "Twinkle, Twinkle Little Star" and "One, Two, Buckle My Shoe."
- Help children learn measurements and fractions by inviting them to help you cook and bake.
- Keep a calendar. This helps children learn names of the days of the week and the number of days in a week, month, and year.
- Play board games, or put together puzzles with your child. These activities help children learn math concepts such as counting, planning ahead, patterns, and special sense.
- Build with blocks, empty boxes, etc., counting as you go along.
- Ask your child to guess how long it will take to do something. Examples include getting dressed and brushing teeth.

How Parents Can Help Their Children Avoid Alcohol and Drugs

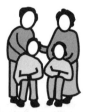 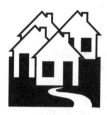 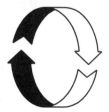  

Parents do not need to feel alone in their fight against drugs. Effective preventative intervention programs are available to schools, families, and communities. Becoming involved is the best way to ensure that strong antidrug policies exist at your child's school. Parents can become involved by doing the following:

♦ **Learn about the school's current policies regarding alcohol and other drugs.**

If no antidrug policy is in place, attend Parent–Teachers' Association or curriculum review meetings, or schedule an interview with the principal to help develop a policy. The policy should specify what constitutes an alcohol, tobacco, or other drug offense; spell out the consequences for failing to follow the rules; and describe procedures for handling violations.

♦ **Become familiar with how drug education is taught in your child's school.**

Are faculty members trained to teach about alcohol, tobacco, and other drug use? Is drug education taught in an age-appropriate manner at each grade level throughout the year or only once during a special week? Is drug education taught only during health class, or do all the teachers incorporate antidrug information into their classes? Is there a parent education component? Is the school's program based on current research?

♦ **Examine the content of the school's drug education program.**

Ask your child to show you any materials distributed during or outside class, and take the opportunity to review them together.

♦ **Find out if your child's school conducts assessments of its drug problem.**

Determine whether these results are used in the antidrug program.

♦ **Ask what happens to children who are caught abusing drugs.**

Does the school offer a list of referrals for students who need special help?

♦ **Request and examine any existing materials.**

Do they contain a clear message that alcohol, tobacco, and other drug use is wrong and harmful? Is the information accurate and up to date?

- ♦ **Investigate whether your school's drug program is evaluated for success.**

  Research indicates that some of the most effective programs emphasize the value of life skills such as coping with anxiety, being assertive, and feeling comfortable socially.

Reclaiming Neighborhoods

Concerned and involved parents can reclaim neighborhoods by doing the following:

- ♦ **Form a community patrol, block association, or Neighborhood Watch.**

  Members can take turns patrolling the block and recording license plate numbers of suspicious cars.

- ♦ **Increase two-way communication with the police.**

  Invite them to neighborhood meetings and keep them informed about suspicious drug activities, which can be reported anonymously.

- ♦ **Make the neighborhood uninviting to drug dealers.**

  Fill the streets with volleyball games, block parties, and other events that make a strong showing of unity to drug dealers.

- ♦ **Call the city Public Works Department for help in cleaning up streets.**

  Blazing lights, litter-free streets, and newly planted flower beds tell drug dealers that residents care about their neighborhood and won't allow drug-related activities to take place there.

- ♦ **Provide positive outlets for the energies of local young people.**

  Unstructured time invites young people to become attracted to drug dealing, an activity that increases the likelihood that they'll become drug users.

- ♦ **Continue to reassure children that you love them and don't want them to use drugs.**

What Parents Can Do if They Think Their Child May Be Taking Drugs

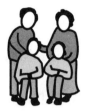 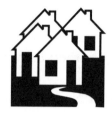 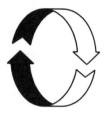 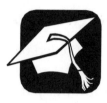 

Parents may find it difficult to identify signs of alcohol and drug abuse. If your child exhibits one or more of the signs listed below, drug abuse may be at the heart of the problem. Signs that your child may be using drugs include the following:

- ◆ She's withdrawn, depressed, tired, and careless about positive grooming.
- ◆ He's hostile and uncooperative, and he frequently breaks curfews.
- ◆ Her relationships with family members have deteriorated.
- ◆ He's hanging around with a new group of friends you don't know.
- ◆ Her grades have slipped, and her school attendance is irregular.
- ◆ He's lost interest in hobbies, sports, and other favorite activities.
- ◆ Her eating or sleeping patterns have changed; she's stays up at night and sleeps during the day.
- ◆ He has a hard time concentrating.
- ◆ Her eyes are red-rimmed and/or her nose is runny in the absence of a cold.
- ◆ Household money has been disappearing.
- ◆ You find rolling papers, small medicine bottles, eye drops, or pipes around the house, in your child's room, or among his personal belongings, including school backpacks and pockets in clothing.

What Parents Can Do

Children are vulnerable to drugs all of their lives, but they are most vulnerable when they leave elementary school and start attending middle school or junior high school. Continue the dialogue on drugs that you began when your child was younger, and stay involved in your child's daily life by encouraging her interests and monitoring her activities. Use the suggestions listed below to significantly decrease the chance of your child becoming involved with drugs. Some of these actions may seem like common sense. Others may meet with resistance from preteens who are striving to achieve independence from their parents. All of the measures listed below are critically important in making sure that your child's life is structured in such a way that drugs have no place in it.

♦ If possible, arrange to have your children looked after and engaged from 3–5 PM.

Encourage them to get involved with youth groups, arts, music, sports, and community service and academic clubs.

♦ Make sure your presence is felt by children who are unattended for periods of time during the day.

Give them a schedule, and set limits on their behavior. Give them household chores to accomplish. Enforce a strict phone-in-to-you policy at a specified time. Leave notes for them around the house. Provide easy-to-find snacks.

♦ Get to know the parents of your child's friends.

Exchange phone numbers and addresses with them. Have everyone agree to forbid each other's children from consuming alcohol, tobacco, and other drugs in their homes, and pledge that you will inform each other if one of you becomes aware of a child who violates this pact.

♦ Call parents whose home is to be used for a party.

Make sure they can assure to your satisfaction that no alcoholic beverages or illegal substances will be dispensed. Don't be afraid to check out the party yourself to see that adult supervision is in place.

♦ Make it easy for your child to leave a place where substances are being used.

Discuss in advance how to contact you or another designated adult to get a ride home. If another adult provides the transportation, be up and available to talk about the incident when your child arrives home.

♦ Set curfews, and enforce them.

Weekend curfews might range from 9:00 pm for a fifth-grade student to 12:30 am for a senior in high school.

♦ Encourage open dialogue with your children about their experience.

Tell your child, "I love you and trust you, but I don't trust the world around you. I need to know what's going on in your life so I can be a good parent to you."

How to Prepare a Checklist for a Meeting with Parents and Guardians

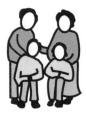 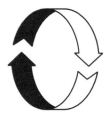   

Teachers and counselors must be prepared for a meeting with parents and guardians. One of the best preparedness checklists comes from the Student Success Program in California.

The mission of the Student Success Team is to create a learning environment that contributes to the achievement, well being, and success of students, parents, teachers, counselors, and administrators. The team process provides for early identification, a collective review, and early intervention planning. Its problem-solving and coordinated approach helps students, families, and school personnel seek positive solutions for maximizing a student's potential.

Review the student's cumulative file and other records, paying particular attention to the following:

☐ History of standardized achievement test data

☐ Hearing and vision screening results and health issues

☐ Past school history, including retention and referral to other programs

☐ History of contacts with the family

Be prepared to present specific background information about the student, including the following:

☐ Strengths (to be built on when developing interventions and modifications)

- Academic (examples include good at math problem solving, likes to read, enjoys art and music, loves to sing, works well on the computer, writes creatively, created an exceptional science project)

- Social/emotional (examples include wants to please adults, chosen by classmates as a friend and/or leader)

- Multiple intelligence characteristics (examples include linguistic, logical–mathematical, bodily–kinesthetic, spatial, musical, interpersonal, intrapersonal)

☐ Interests (including preferences for reading and writing topics, science and math themes, projects, etc.)

☐ Academic functioning in reading, oral language, written language, and math (bring curriculum-based data to show levels)

☐ Amount and quality of class work and homework (bring recent work samples)

Be ready to discuss the following:

☐ Your basic concern(s) (academic, behavior, social–emotional, health, etc.)

☐ Desired student outcomes (the improvements you would like to see as concrete outcomes, such as better attendance, increased reading or math skills, improved ability to work with and get along with peers, ability to follow classroom or playground rules)

☐ Strategies and modifications you have tried

☐ Analysis of classroom environment

☐ Efforts to work with the family to resolve your concerns

Bring the following to the meeting:

☐ Student's cumulative file

☐ Recent work samples that reflect both strengths and areas of concern

☐ In-class assessments that show academic levels

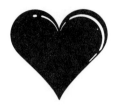

Early Childhood Education

Interventions that take place between birth and three years demonstrate that providing a child with educational enrichment can modify IQ. The most effective way to decrease the number of children who will ultimately drop out is to provide the best possible classroom instruction from the beginning of the school experience. Tools in this module include:

"How to Help Children Develop Listening and Speaking Skills," adapted from "Teaching Our Youngest," United States Department of Education and United States Department of Health and Human Services Early Childhood–Head Start Task Force, Washington, D.C., 2002.

"How to Build Children's Background Knowledge and Thinking Skills," adapted from "Teaching Our Youngest," United States Department of Education and United States Department of Health and Human Services Early Childhood–Head Start Task Force, Washington, D.C., 2002.

"How to Help Young Children Learn About Numbers," adapted from "Teaching Our Youngest," United States Department of Education and United States Department of Health and Human Services Early Childhood–Head Start Task Force, Washington, D.C., 2002.

How to Help Children Develop Listening and Speaking Skills

 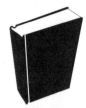 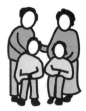  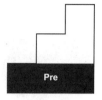

Frequently, we assume that children know how to listen and speak. Realistically, these skills need to be taught. To gain valuable language skills, children must be instructed in how to listen to teachers, parents, and peers.

It is important for young children to be able to do the following:

- ♦ Listen carefully for different purposes, such as to get information or for enjoyment.
- ♦ Use spoken language for a variety of purposes.
- ♦ Follow and give simple directions and instructions.
- ♦ Ask and answer questions.
- ♦ Use appropriate volume and speed when speaking.
- ♦ Participate in discussions and follow the rules of polite conversation, such as staying on a topic and taking turns.
- ♦ Use language to express their feelings and ideas.

It is important for teachers to do the following:

- ♦ Ask open-ended questions, which invite children to expand on their answers.
- ♦ Present new words to children so they can expand their vocabularies.
- ♦ Respond to questions, and let children take the conversational lead.
- ♦ Respond to children's questions so they can build their language skills.

Here are some things parents can do to help develop their children's listening and speaking skills:

- ♦ Engage children in conversation throughout the day.
- ♦ When reading aloud, encourage children to predict what will happen in the story, to comment on the story, and to make connections between the story and their personal experiences.
- ♦ Play games that focus children's attention on the importance of listening carefully.
- ♦ Gently reinforce the rules of good listening and speaking throughout the day.
- ♦ Capitalize on routine opportunities to have children follow or give directions.

How to Build Children's Background Knowledge and Thinking Skills

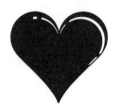 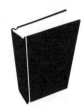 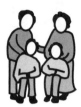  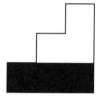

"The more children know about their world, the easier it is for them to read and learn when they get to school. Teachers have an important role to play in helping children learn new information, ideas, and vocabulary and learn how to use this knowledge to become full participants in their own learning. Teachers, parents and child-care givers can help children to connect new information and ideas to what they already know and understand."

From: *Teaching Our Youngest,* United States Department of Education

It is important for young children to be able to do the following:

♦ Know what things are and how they work.

♦ Learn information about the world around them.

♦ Expand their use of language and develop their vocabulary.

♦ Develop their ability to figure things out and to solve problems.

Here are some things that teachers of young children can do to help them build knowledge:

♦ Provide them with opportunities to develop concepts by exploring and working with familiar classroom equipment and materials in a variety of ways.

  • Children learn about substances and changes in substances by cooking.

  • Children learn about plants by planting seeds and taking care of the growing plants.

  • Children learn about social situations and interactions through real interactions and dramatic play.

♦ Share informational books.

  • Children enjoy learning about their world. They enjoy looking at books about things of interest to them, perhaps how plants grow, how baby animals develop, or how vehicles carry people and things. Fortunately, many wonderful informational books are available that have spectacular photographs or illustrations and descriptions that children can easily understand.

♦ Teach the children new words and concepts.

- Explain new vocabulary in the books that you read with children. Teach them and name all of the things in the classroom. In everyday talk with children, introduce words and concepts that they may not know, such as "beauty" or "fairness."

♦ Have children write, draw, build, and engage in dramatic play.
- These experiences will help children incorporate what they are learning into what they already know.

♦ Take children on field trips.
- Whenever children go someplace, especially someplace new to them, they can learn something. Even if it is just a walk around the block, children can learn something new if you talk with them. Point out things they might not normally notice. Explain events that are taking place. Answer questions they pose, and praise them for looking and learning. Before you go to a place the children have never been, such as a zoo or a museum, discuss what they will be seeing and learning. After the trip, invite the children talk about their experiences.

♦ Provide a variety of materials for your children to explore. Examples include wire, cardboard, water, tubing, and tissue paper.

♦ Invite visitors to your classroom.
- Classroom visitors can teach your children a great deal. They can bring interesting objects or animals to talk about with the children. Visitors can describe their jobs or hobbies, show pictures of faraway places they have visited, or tell stories about life when they were young.

How to Help Young Children Learn About Numbers

 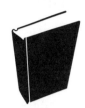 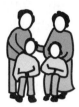  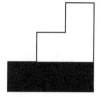

"Many children enter preschool with some knowledge of numbers and counting. They can count five to ten objects accurately and can also read some numbers. But many other children have not developed this knowledge. These children, in particular, need many opportunities to learn the words for numbers, to count things, and to learn to read and write numbers."

From: *Teaching Our Youngest,* United States Department of Education

Parents and teachers can help children learn about numbers and counting in many ways, including these informal suggestions:

- ◆ Make pointing to and counting objects part of your daily routine.
- ◆ While you point and count, ask the children to count with you and then without you. Children need to hear and practice things often to learn them.
- ◆ Help children learn to answer the "how many?" question.
- ◆ Children like to point to and count their fingers, legs, and ears. Help them do this.
- ◆ Using different types of macaroni, encourage children to sort the different types and then count them.
- ◆ Give children rulers, and let them measure different things around the room.

Teach children counting songs and rhymes. You can play counting games using many different actions, such as jumping and clapping. As children learn more number words, they can count more actions.

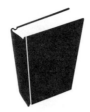

Reading and Writing Programs

Early interventions to help low-achieving students recognize that focusing on reading and writing skills are the foundation for effective learning in all subjects. Tools in this module include:

"How to Design an Elementary School Writing System," developed by Marlane Parra and Debbie Schwebke, Mesilla Park Elementary School, 3101 Bowman Street, Las Cruces, New Mexico; marlane@zianet.com.

"How to Measure a Student's Skill in Talking and Understanding Sentences—Kindergarten," developed by Marlane Parra and Debbie Schwebke, Mesilla Park Elementary School, 3101 Bowman Street, Las Cruces, New Mexico; marlane@zianet.com.

"Writing Rubric: Sentences—First Grade," developed by Marlane Parra and Debbie Schwebke, Mesilla Park Elementary School, 3101 Bowman Street, Las Cruces, New Mexico; marlane@zianet.com.

"Writing Rubric: Paragraphs—Second Grade," developed by Marlane Parra and Debbie Schwebke, Mesilla Park Elementary School, 3101 Bowman Street, Las Cruces, New Mexico; marlane@zianet.com.

"The Funnel Plan for Writing Paragraphs—Second Grade," developed by Marlane Parra and Debbie Schwebke, Mesilla Park Elementary School, 3101 Bowman Street, Las Cruces, New Mexico; marlane@zianet.com.

"How to Teach Students to Write a Paragraph—Second Grade," developed by Marlane Parra and Debbie Schwebke, Mesilla Park Elementary School, 3101 Bowman Street, Las Cruces, New Mexico; marlane@zianet.com.

"Writing Rubric—Third Grade," developed by Marlane Parra and Debbie Schwebke, Mesilla Park Elementary School, 3101 Bowman Street, Las Cruces, New Mexico; marlane @zianet.com.

How to Design an Elementary School Writing System

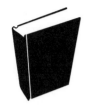  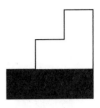

Reading and writing programs are inherent within all successful learning systems. Two elementary school teachers in Las Cruces, New Mexico, have developed a series of rubrics (below) to measure the success of their reading program.

Design for an elementary school writing program

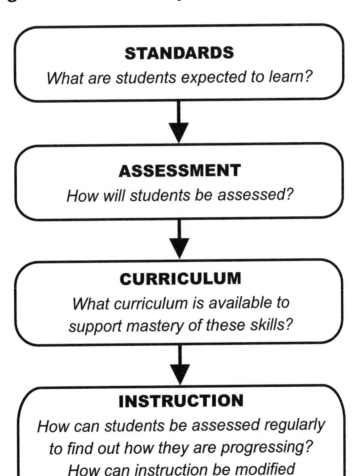

STANDARDS
What are students expected to learn?

ASSESSMENT
How will students be assessed?

CURRICULUM
What curriculum is available to support mastery of these skills?

INSTRUCTION
How can students be assessed regularly to find out how they are progressing? How can instruction be modified continually to meet their dynamic needs?

How to Measure a Student's Skill in Talking and Understanding Sentences—Kindergarten

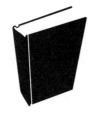  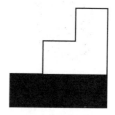

Two elementary teachers in Las Cruces, New Mexico, have developed a series of rubrics to measure the success of their reading program (below). Rubrics form a key element in determining the expertise of students.

Rubric for assessing a kindergarten student's skill in talking and understanding sentences

Student: _____

Class: _____

Date: _____

Sentence Formation

3   Can say a complete, grammatically correct sentence about a given picture or topic.

2   Can say a complete, grammatically correct sentence, but not about assigned picture or topic.

1   Cannot say a complete, grammatically correct sentence about assigned picture or topic.

Sentence Awareness

3   Can point to entire sentence in text (from initial word through final word) AND state that a sentence tells a complete thought.

2   Can point to an entire sentence in text (from initial word through final word) OR state that a sentence tells a complete thought.

1   Cannot point to entire sentence in text (from initial word through final word) OR state that a sentence tells a complete thought.

Mechanics (Capitalization, Punctuation, and Spelling)

3   Can point to initial capital letter AND ending punctuation in text.

2   Can point to initial capital letter OR ending punctuation in text.

1   Cannot point to initial capital letter OR ending punctuation in text.

Writing Rubric: Sentences—First Grade

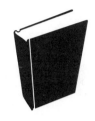  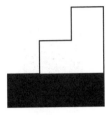

Two elementary teachers in Las Cruces, New Mexico, have developed a series of rubrics to measure the success of their reading program (below).

Rubric for assessing a first-grader's ability to understand and form sentences

Student: _____

Class: _____

Date: _____

Analytic Scores

Sentence Formation

3   Sentence is complete and about assigned topic.

2   Sentence is complete but not about assigned topic.

1   Sentence is not complete.

Mechanics (capitalization, punctuation, spelling)

3   Has beginning capital letter and correct ending punctuation.

2   Has beginning capital letter OR correct ending punctuation.

1   Does not have a beginning capital letter AND does not have ending punctuation.

Word Usage

3   All correct word usage AND used at least one detail word

2   No more than one error in word usage

1   More than one error in word usage

Writing Rubric: Paragraphs—Second Grade

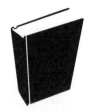  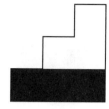

Two elementary teachers in Las Cruces, New Mexico, have developed a series of rubrics to measure the success of their reading program (below).]

Rubric for assessing a second-grader's ability to understand and form paragraphs

Student: _____

Class: _____

Date: _____

Analytic Scores

Sentence Formation

3   All sentences are complete

2   Only one incomplete sentence (or 80% of sentences are complete)

1   Less than 80% of sentences are complete

Mechanics (capitalization, punctuation, spelling)

3   All sentences start with a capital letter; all sentences have ending punctuation; first sentence is indented; fewer than two spelling errors

2   Less than 10% punctuation and capitalization errors; may not have indention; three to six spelling errors

1   Less than 10% punctuation and capitalization errors; may not have indention; more than six spelling errors

Word Usage

3   Descriptive/detail words are used; few or no problems with subject/verb agreement; employs correct pronouns, possessives, and verb forms

2   Ordinary, everyday vocabulary; some problems with subject/verb agreement; some errors in correct pronouns, possessives, and verb forms.

1   Limited vocabulary; many problems with subject/verb agreement; many errors in correct pronouns, possessives, and verb forms.

Development (Must Have Five or More Sentences)

3   Has topic sentence and three or more supporting sentences and closing sentence.

2   Has topic sentence and three or more supporting sentences OR no closing sentence.

1   No topic sentence OR not all sentences related to topic.

The Funnel Plan for Writing Paragraphs—Second Grade

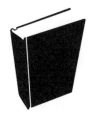  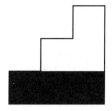

Below is the Funnel plan to teach second-grade students how to write a paragraph.

Funnel plan for teaching second-grade students how to write paragraphs.

Sentence One States:

1. What I'm talking about AND

2. Three describing words or ideas

Sentence Two Tells:

About the first descriptive word or idea

Sentence Three Tells:

About the second descriptive word or idea

Sentence Four Tells:

About the third descriptive word or idea

Sentence Five Restates:

The first sentence but with different words I found in the thesaurus

How to Teach Students to Write a Paragraph—Second Grade

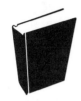 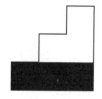

Two elementary teachers in Las Cruces, New Mexico, have developed a series of rubrics to measure the success of their reading program (below).

How to teach second-grade students to write a paragraph

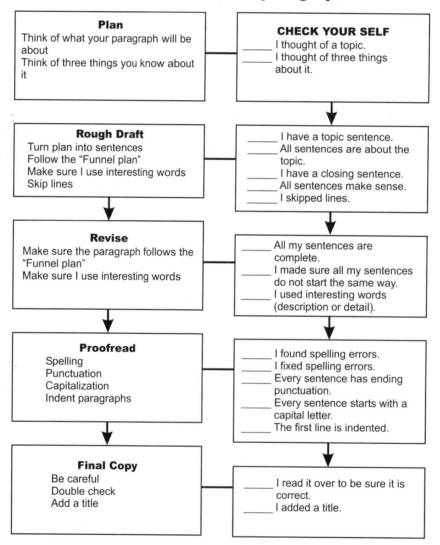

Plan
Think of what your paragraph will be about
Think of three things you know about it

CHECK YOUR SELF
_____ I thought of a topic.
_____ I thought of three things about it.

Rough Draft
Turn plan into sentences
Follow the "Funnel plan"
Make sure I use interesting words
Skip lines

_____ I have a topic sentence.
_____ All sentences are about the topic.
_____ I have a closing sentence.
_____ All sentences make sense.
_____ I skipped lines.

Revise
Make sure the paragraph follows the "Funnel plan"
Make sure I use interesting words

_____ All my sentences are complete.
_____ I made sure all my sentences do not start the same way.
_____ I used interesting words (description or detail).

Proofread
Spelling
Punctuation
Capitalization
Indent paragraphs

_____ I found spelling errors.
_____ I fixed spelling errors.
_____ Every sentence has ending punctuation.
_____ Every sentence starts with a capital letter.
_____ The first line is indented.

Final Copy
Be careful
Double check
Add a title

_____ I read it over to be sure it is correct.
_____ I added a title.

Writing Rubric—Third Grade

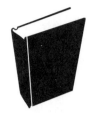  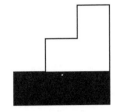

Two elementary teachers in Las Cruces, New Mexico, have developed a series of rubrics to measure the success of their reading program (below).

Rubric for assessing the ability of third-grade students to write.

Student: _____

Class: _____

Writing Mode   Narrative   Expository

Analytic Scores

Sentence Formation

3 Complete sentences with a variety of length and type; reads smoothly together

2 Basically good sentence structure with occasional confusing constructions; few run-on or fragment sentences; most sentences start the same

1 Simple, short sentences; many run-on or fragment sentences

Mechanics (capitalization, punctuation, spelling)

3 Good punctuation and capitalization (few errors); no or few spelling errors.

2 Some punctuation and capitalization errors; several spelling errors

1 Many capitalization and punctuation errors; several spelling errors

Word Usage

3 Imaginative use of words; few or no problems with subject/verb agreement; correct pronouns, possessives, and verb forms

2 Ordinary, everyday language; some problems with subject/verb agreement; some errors in pronouns, possessives, and verb forms

1 Limited vocabulary; many problems with subject/verb agreement; many errors in pronouns, possessives, and verb forms

Development (narrative)	OR	*Development (expository)*
3 Follows main idea to end; organized; good description; problem matches solution		3 Follows main idea; many facts and details; well organized
2 Has problem and solution; development not clear; not all events relate clearly		2 Specific facts and details but unevenly used or poorly organized; poor transitions
1 No problem and solution		1 Few facts and details; sketchy, vague, or confusing

Mentoring and Tutoring

Mentoring is a one-to-one caring, supportive relationship between a mentor and a mentee that is based on trust. Tutoring, also a one-to-one activity, focuses on academics and is an effective way to address specific needs such as reading, writing, or math competencies. Tools in this module include:

"What Exactly Does a Mentor Do?" adapted from *Everyday Heroes: A Guidebook for Mentors* by Jim Kavanaugh, Ph.D., based on the Wise Men and Women Mentorship Program, Kenneth J. Carson, Sr., Founder and Director; contributed by Jim Kavanaugh, Ph.D., and Kenneth J. Carson

"Questions a Mentor Should Ask Himself or Herself" adapted from *Everyday Heroes: A Guidebook for Mentors* by Jim Kavanaugh, Ph.D., based on the Wise Men and Women Mentorship Program, Kenneth J. Carson, Sr., Founder and Director; contributed by Jim Kavanaugh, Ph.D., and Kenneth J. Carson

"How to Establish a Good Mentoring Relationship," adapted from *Everyday Heroes: A Guidebook for Mentors* by Jim Kavanaugh, Ph.D., based on the Wise Men and Women Mentorship Program, Kenneth J. Carson, Sr., Founder and Director; contributed by Jim Kavanaugh, Ph.D., and Kenneth J. Carson

"Your First Day As a Mentor," adapted from *Everyday Heroes: A Guidebook for Mentors* by Jim Kavanaugh, Ph.D., based on the Wise Men and Women Mentorship Program, Kenneth J. Carson, Sr., Founder and Director; contributed by Jim Kavanaugh, Ph.D., and Kenneth J. Carson

What Exactly Does a Mentor Do?

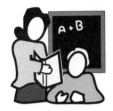   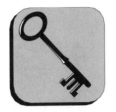 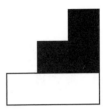

Although mentoring is not a problem-focused or solution-oriented endeavor, such as counseling or psychotherapy, it can help children to lead a healthy life. In fact, scientific research suggests that one of the most effect ingredients in all forms of counseling is the unconditional regard of one person for another.

The most important outcomes of mentoring are the following:

♦ Mentors make children feel unique, special, and good about themselves.

♦ Mentors provide children with consistent and unconditional support, which helps them feel safe in the world.

♦ Mentors allow children to become attached to them, which increases the child's ability to form nurturing relationships with others.

♦ Mentors model positive values, attitudes, and behaviors, which encourages children's ability to do likewise.

♦ Mentors help children to discover solutions to their problems, which increases their sense of confidence and self-reliance.

♦ Mentors help children to look beyond today to see tomorrow' possibilities, which increases their sense of hope and raises their expectations for the future.

Mentoring relationships foster the following:

♦ Self-esteem

♦ Positive relationships

♦ Sense of hope

♦ Positive social orientation

♦ Feeling of safety

♦ High self-expectations

Questions a Mentor Should Ask Himself or Herself

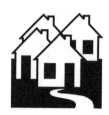

Each potential mentor needs to look inward and give some serious thought to the following questions:

- Why am I doing this? Do I have the right motivation for this work?
- Do I genuinely like children? Will I really enjoy this?
- Are there some type of children with whom I might have difficulty? If so, what types and why?
- Do I have the openness to enter a child's world; the understanding to accept his or her background; and the patience to go at his or her pace?
- Do I believe that children's lives can improve and that one person can make a difference?
- Do I truly have the time for this? Will it throw the rest of my life into imbalance?
- Do I have the support of my significant others to do this? Will they object to this extra responsibility?
- Can I really mentor an entire school year? Am I successfully managing the other commitments in my life?
- What personal strengths and interests can I bring to the mentoring relationship?
- What kinds of support and assistance will I need to be the most effective mentor I can be?
- Am I receptive to new ideas and ways of doing things? Can I learn and change?
- Can I work cooperatively with others, or would I rather do things on my own?
- Overall, does mentoring fit well with my life and my personality? Should I be a mentor?

How to Establish a
Good Mentoring Relationship

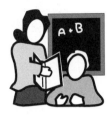  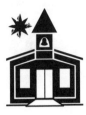 

Mentoring is a unique relationship that does not come naturally to people. People must be trained how to act both as mentors and mentees. Some begin this relationship with apprehension and concern. Many mentors enter the relationship without a clear understanding of their role or how to achieve it. Many mentees experience great curiosity about being mentored and have many questions.

Preparation and training increase the likelihood of a successful mentor/mentee relationship. The following information supports this likelihood:

A good mentoring relationship . . .

- ◆ requires informed parental consent,
- ◆ involves frequent and regular contact,
- ◆ requires at least a one-year commitment,
- ◆ focuses solely on the needs of the child,
- ◆ protects the rights and dignity of the child,
- ◆ respects cultural differences,
- ◆ is guided by the child's interests,
- ◆ relies in large part on active listening by the mentor,
- ◆ employs communication at the child's level,
- ◆ generates a sense of warmth and openness,
- ◆ explores themes important to daily life,
- ◆ builds on the child's strengths,
- ◆ supports the best of human values, and
- ◆ reflects the best of human values.

Your First Day As a Mentor

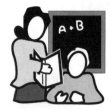   

How mentors act the first day "on the job" frequently determines the student's and the school's perception of them. A leading mentorship program, the Wise Men and Women Mentorship Program, advocates the advice listed below.

- Dress appropriately, i.e., not too informally yet not overly formal.
- Greet children whom you meet or pass in a friendly manner.
- Keep an open mind, and do not appear judgmental.
- Go directly to the appropriate office. Your school contact will most likely be the school counselor.
- Take some time to get to know the counselor. He will become an important resource.
- Do not ask the counselor for more information than necessary about your mentee, e.g., name, age, class level, and basic concerns.
- Do everything you can to eventually meet the school principal. She should know who you are and what you do.
- Do not be too surprised about the room you are given. Available space in a school is frequently a coveted item.
- If the counselor forgets to offer, ask him to introduce you to your mentee.

Remember that good mentorship depends on the quality of your presence. From the moment you walk onto school grounds, you want to establish a climate of openness, caring, and safety.

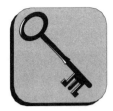

Service Learning

Service learning connects meaningful community service experiences with academic learning. This method for teaching and learning promotes personal and social growth, career development, and civic responsibility and can be a powerful vehicle for effective school reform at all grade levels. The tool in this module is:

"How to Track and Evaluate a Service Learning Program," adapted from American YouthWorks Charter School, Lois Myers, Curriculum Specialist, Austin TX 78701; (512) 236-6150

How to Track and Evaluate a Service Learning Program

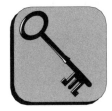 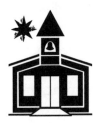 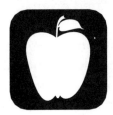 

American YouthWorks Charter School in Austin, Texas, incorporates service learning (below) across disciplines and distributes credits. Areas tracked include research skills, communication skills, evaluation skills, reflection, and portfolios.

Why is service learning effective? Participants develop relationships with program facilitators, gain a sense of autonomy, and feel more competent in their relationships with peers and adults. They also feel empowered by the knowledge that they can make a difference in the lives of others.

Service Learning Flow Chart: The Route of the Master Tracking Sheet

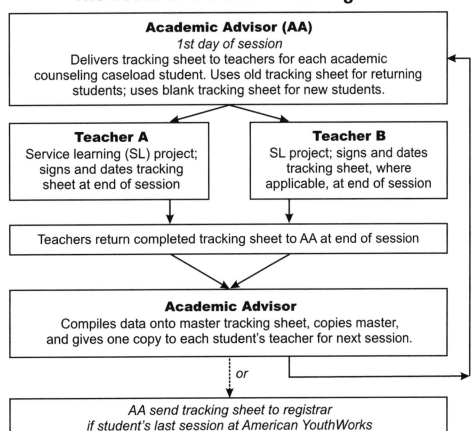

In Other Words...

♦ Academic advisors (AAs) make two copies of each student's service learning (SL) master tracking sheet (p. 39). The academic advisor uses an updated tracking sheet for returning students and a blank tracking sheet for new students. The updated original tracking sheet is kept in the student's folder.

♦ The academic advisor distributes one copy of the tracking sheet to each teacher of their advising caseload students.

♦ The teacher facilitates all or part of a service learning project, and the student takes an active role in one or more project objectives.

♦ At end of session, the teacher initials and dates the tracking sheet where applicable for each student and returns the sheets to the academic advisor.

♦ The academic advisor compiles the new information on the master tracking sheet in the student's folder and makes two copies of master tracking sheet to give to the next session's teachers.

♦ This process is continued every session until the student graduates.

♦ When the student graduates, the academic advisor sends the completed tracking sheet to the registrar, who then assigns credit and signs and dates the tracking sheet.

American YouthWorks Charter School Service Learning Tracking Sheet

Student name [ ]

Earliest graduation date [ ]

Service Learning (SL) projects & dates:

1 [ ]   2 [ ]   3 [ ]   4 [ ]

5 [ ]   6 [ ]   7 [ ]   8 [ ]

SL Objectives	Fall 2002 Teacher Initial & Date	Winter 2002 Teacher Initial & Date	Spring 2003 Teacher Initial & Date	Sum. 2003 Teacher Initial & Date	Fall 2003 Teacher Initial & Date	Winter 2003 Teacher Initial & Date	Spring 2004 Teacher Initial & Date	Sum. 2004 Teacher Initial & Date
Step 1 Research Community Need								
Phone calls, interviews, Internet search, local sources								
Surveys								
Focus groups								
Field trips								
Evaluate research and identify project								
Reflection (formative)								
Other (specify)								
Step 2 Design and Prepare SL Project								
Define project goal								
Identify asks, resources, timeline, responsibilities								
Communicate with project partners and participants								
Create evaluation form								
Reflection (formative)								
Other (specify)								

SL Objectives	Fall 2002 Teacher Initial & Date	Winter 2002 Teacher Initial & Date	Spring 2003 Teacher Initial & Date	Sum. 2003 Teacher Initial & Date	Fall 2003 Teacher Initial & Date	Winter 2003 Teacher Initial & Date	Spring 2004 Teacher Initial & Date	Sum. 2004 Teacher Initial & Date

Step 3   *Implement Project*

Carry out design plan	☐	☐	☐	☐	☐	☐	☐	☐
Reflection (formative)	☐	☐	☐	☐	☐	☐	☐	☐
Other (specify)	☐	☐	☐	☐	☐	☐	☐	☐

Step 4   *Reflection on SL Project (Summative)*

Discussion, journals, essays	☐	☐	☐	☐	☐	☐	☐	☐
Project portfolio	☐	☐	☐	☐	☐	☐	☐	☐
Interview with community volunteer role models	☐	☐	☐	☐	☐	☐	☐	☐
Other (specify)	☐	☐	☐	☐	☐	☐	☐	☐

*For credit approval, students must have a minimum of three completed check boxes in each SL objective.

*Students who are enrolled for one session before graduation must have one completed checkbox in each SL objective.

SL credit will be assigned on the final transcript!

☑ Approved for .5 credit: _____   _____
                           Registrar's signature   Date

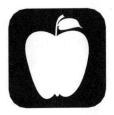

Alternative Schooling

Alternative schooling provides potential dropouts with a variety of options that can lead to graduation, with programs paying special attention to the students' individual social needs and the academic requirements for a high school diploma. Tools in this module include:

"What Services Should Alternative Schools Offer?" donated by Project Transition, Bryan Station Traditional High School, 1866 Edgeworth Drive, Lexington, Kentucky 40505, (859) 299-3392; written by Lonnie, L. Leland, Program Coordinator, and Becky LaVey, M.S.W., Program Social Worker.

"Developing An Alternative Education Program Standard," developed by the Kentucky Department of Education, 500 Mero Street, Frankfort, Kentucky 40601, (502) 564-3678; contributed by Leon Swarts, Student, Family, and Community Support Services.

"How to Align Alternative Education Programs with Standards—Review Summary," developed by the Kentucky Department of Education, 500 Mero Street, Frankfort, Kentucky 40601, (502) 564-3678; contributed by Leon Swarts, Student, Family, and Community Support Services.

"How to Monitor Academic Performance," donated by Project Transition, Bryan Station Traditional High School, 1866 Edgeworth Drive, Lexington, Kentucky 40505, (859) 299-3392; written by Lonnie L. Leland, Program Coordinator, and Becky LaVey, M.S.W., Program Social Worker.

"How to Hire an Alternative Education Teacher," adapted from the Success Academy Shadowing Intervention Program, Pickerington High School, 300 Opportunity Way, Pickerington, Ohio 43147, (614) 833-3025; Mike Smith, Principal, Renee Riddle, Shadowing and Intervention Teacher, and Julie Brunner, Guidance Counselor; julie_brunner@ fc.pickerington.k12.oh.us and www.pickerington.k12.oh.us, 614-833-3038.

"How to Hire an Instructional Intervention Assistant," adapted from the Success Academy Shadowing Intervention Program, Pickerington High School, 300 Opportunity Way, Pickerington, Ohio, 43147, (614) 833-3025; Mike Smith, Principal, Renee Riddle, Shadowing and Intervention Teacher, and Julie

"How to Monitor Student Behavior Using a Checklist," adapted from the San Jose Unified School District, Student Services and Guidance, 855 Lenzen Avenue, San Jose, California 95126, (408) 535-6197.

"Entering Middle And High School Student Self-Assessment," adapted from the Success Academy Shadowing Intervention Program, Pickerington High School, 300 Opportunity Way, Pickerington, Ohio, 43147, (614) 833-3025; Jim Thompson, Renee Riddle, Shadowing and Intervention Teacher, and Julie Brunner, Guidance Counselor; julie_brunner@fc.pickerington.k12.oh.us and www.pickerington.k12.oh.us, 614-833-3038.

What Services Should Alternative Schools Offer?

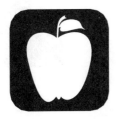 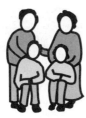   

Project Transition's unique approach is to team educators with social workers who work closely with students and their parents. The systemic approach of the program addresses areas of improving academic and interpersonal skills as well as self-esteem. In addition, it provides students with a career vocational and assessment program. Part-time jobs are provided by businesses that cooperate with the program. The program has shown an overall 55% increase in classes passed and a 63% decrease in absences. The student group has resulted in a decrease in number of suspensions and days suspended of more than 90%. Project Transition has been awarded the Crystal Star of Excellence Award by the National Dropout Prevention Center.

Project Transition encompasses the following:

- Daily monitoring of student attendance and follow-up calls to the parent or guardian during morning hours
- Contact with each student every morning to gain awareness of student needs
- Teacher assistance
- Individual student tutoring
- Student involvement in various statewide and countywide competitions
- Liaison between home and school
- Liaison between school and outside service agencies (public and private)
- Conferences and interventions with students
- Educational and career-shadowing experiences
- Career assessment and learning styles testing
- Student support groups (teen parents, parents of teens, grief support, self-esteem, conflict management)
- Training in study skills
- Crisis intervention
- Incentives and rewards for academic improvement and success
- Academic monitoring sheets
- Parent counseling and home contacts
- Scholarship program

Developing an Alternative Education Program Standard

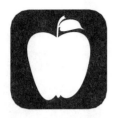 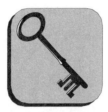   

The Kentucky State Department of Education has developed a set of standards to judge the efficiency and effectiveness of alternative education programs. These standards can also be used to evaluate a whole host of programs and schools.

- *Effective planning:* Supervisors, teachers, and other staff take into consideration facility operations and management staff members; staff member assignment and support; and student entry and exit criteria, classroom placement, and support.

- *Professional development:* Staff members are given opportunities to develop high-quality academic and/or behavior management skills.

- *Academic practices:* Teachers set high standards for all students, provide support, adjust curriculum, modify instruction, and use a variety of assessment strategies to meet individual student needs.

- *Behavior management practices:* All program staff members use individual needs assessment data to identify interventions and measure specific individual student outcomes (attendance, grades, violations, etc.).

- *Program collaboration:* Staff members access internal district social services, psychological services, exceptional education programs, and resources to provide targeted and intensive support to students and families.

- *Leadership:* Program supervisors and central office administrators work collaboratively with staff members, students, families, and communities to develop, implement, and evaluate program effectiveness.

- *Parent involvement:* Staff work with parents and/or guardians to develop communication and provide advisory, education, and support opportunities.

- *Community involvement:* Staff members access external community service agencies, business and industry, faith-based organizations, law enforcement, etc., to provide targeted and intensive support to students and families.

- *Culture and climate:* The program's mission statement, goals, objectives, belief system, rules, and routines are universally accepted and practiced consistently by all staff members.

- *Student support services:* Counseling, social services, and health assistance are available for all students on a regular basis.

- *Equity and diversity:* Physical, cultural, socioeconomic, racial, and gender differences among staff and students are considered before all program decisions are made.

How to Align Alternative Education Programs with Standards: Review Summary

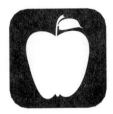 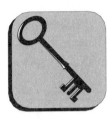 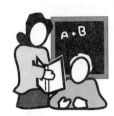  

The Kentucky State Department of Education has developed a set of standards to judge the efficiency and effectiveness of alternative education programs. These standards can be used to evaluate a whole host of programs and schools.

Effective Planning

- ◆ *Standard:* Supervisors, teachers, and other staff take into consideration facility operations and management staff members; staff member assignment and support; and student entry and exit criteria, classroom placement, and support.
- ◆ *Indicators:* yes/no

  _____ Student, academic, social, and behavioral needs
  _____ Academic practices (e.g., curriculum, instruction, and assessment)
  _____ School structure, safety, and location
  _____ Staff and student school calendars
  _____ Low student-to-staff ratios (e.g., 10:1, 12:1, 15:1)
  _____ Materials, supplies, and equipment
  _____ Technology
  _____ Transportation
  _____ Food services

Notes: _____

_____

- ◆ *Standard subtotal* (circle one): Low ➔ High

  1   2   3   4   5

Professional Development

- *Standard:* Staff members are given opportunities to develop high-quality academic and/or behavior management skills.
- *Indicators:* yes/no
  - _____ Long-term strategic program plan
  - _____ Individual staff growth plans
  - _____ Coaching, mentoring, and clinical supervision
  - _____ Attend conferences, retreats, and seminars
  - _____ Participate in workshops, institutes, and seminars

Notes: _____

_____

_____

- *Standard subtotal* (circle one): Low ➜ High

      1   2   3   4   5

Academic Practices

Curriculum

- *Standard for Curriculum:* Based on grade level, functional level, learning styles, multiple intelligences, emotional intelligence, and behavior management needs.
- *Indicators:* yes/no
  - _____ Core content
  - _____ Program of studies
  - _____ Career pathways
  - _____ District curriculum
  - _____ Life skills
  - _____ Social skills
  - _____ Vocational programs
  - _____ Integration
  - _____ Mapping and organizing

Notes: _____

_____

_____

- *Standard subtotal* (circle one): Low ➜ High

      1   2   3   4   5

Instruction

- *Standard for Instruction:* Teachers provide high-quality diagnostic instruction that has value, meaning, and relevance for students.
- *Indicators:* yes/no
  - _____ Highly structured classroom
  - _____ Direct instruction
  - _____ Cooperative learning

_____ Creative development
_____ Individual study and small groups
_____ Behavior management needs
_____ Individual student intelligences and learning styles
_____ Social skills (e.g., anger management, conflict resolution, and problem solving)

Notes: _____

_____

_____

♦ *Standard subtotal* (circle one): Low ➜ High

         1   2   3   4   5

Assessment

♦ *Standard for Assessment:* Teachers and support staff members use multiple assessment strategies to measure student achievement and social and behavioral skills.

♦ *Indicators:* yes/no

_____ Authentic
_____ Performance-based
_____ Standards mastery
_____ Portfolios
_____ Projects
_____ Hands-on
_____ Limited objective testing (e.g., multiple choice, fill-in, etc.)
_____ Behavior scales, social rating scales, learning styles, intelligence surveys

Notes: _____

_____

_____

♦ *Standard subtotal* (circle one): Low ➜ High

         1   2   3   4   5

Behavior Management Practices

♦ *Standard:* All program staff members use individual needs assessment data to identify interventions and measure specific individual student outcomes (attendance, grades, violations, etc.).

♦ *Indicators:* yes/no

_____ Identify causes of behavior
_____ Identify what "keeps students going"
_____ Identify positive replacement behaviors
_____ Interview and involve the student and parents
_____ Uses multicomponent strategies
_____ Use level and point systems

_____ Self-management skills are taught
_____ Use high rates of positive reinforcement

Notes: _____

_____

_____

♦ *Standard subtotal* (circle one): Low ➔ High

1   2   3   4   5

Program Collaboration

♦ *Standard:* Staff members access internal district social services, psychological services, exceptional education programs, and resources to provide targeted and intensive support to students and families.

♦ *Indicators:* yes/no

_____ Family and parents or guardians (e.g., training, monitoring, and coordination)
_____ Community agencies
_____ Law enforcement
_____ Businesses
_____ Service agencies
_____ Speakers, mentors, and community role models
_____ Other schools and districts
_____ Other service providers

Notes: _____

_____

_____

♦ *Standard subtotal* (circle one): Low ➔ High

1   2   3   4   5

Leadership

♦ *Standard:* Program supervisors and central office administrators work collaboratively with staff members, students, families, and communities to develop, implement, and evaluate program effectiveness.

♦ *Indicators:* yes/no

_____ Regulate policies
_____ Establish procedures
_____ Interpret guidelines
_____ Solve problems
_____ Provide consistency and follow-up on all issues
_____ Involve staff in decisions
_____ Facilitate communication
_____ Create a positive culture and climate
_____ Reinforce program mission, beliefs, goals, rules, and routines

Notes: _____

_____

_____

♦ *Standard subtotal* (circle one): Low ➜ High

          1   2   3   4   5

Parent Involvement

♦ *Standard:* Staff members work with parents and/or guardians to develop communication and provide advisory, education, and support opportunities.

♦ *Indicators:* yes/no

_____ Continuous interaction between families and school promotes programs and services for students

_____ Timely information regarding student academic and nonacademic performance available (e.g., program report cards and progress reports)

_____ Families involved in significant ways to support student learning (e.g., assisting with homework, reviewing student work, and attending conferences)

_____ Parents and guardians welcome and assistance sought

_____ Parent advisory group

_____ Opportunities available for parent program education and training

Notes: _____

_____

_____

♦ *Standard subtotal* (circle one): Low ➜High

          1   2   3   4   5

Community Involvement

♦ *Standard:* Staff members access external community service agencies, business and industry, faith-based organizations, law enforcement, etc., to provide targeted and intensive support to students and families.

♦ *Indicators:* yes/no

_____ School, families, and communities are active partners in the educational process

_____ Partnerships formed between school and community to support programs and services

_____ Community advisory committee makes program and service recommendations

_____ Opportunities for students to engage in community-based learning activities (e.g., mentoring, career information, job shadowing, etc.)

Notes: _____

_____

_____

♦ *Standard subtotal* (circle one): Low ➜ High

          1   2   3   4   5

Culture and Climate

- *Standard:* The program's mission statement, goals, objectives, belief system, rules, and routines are universally accepted and practiced consistently by all staff members.
- *Indicators:* yes/no
  - _____ Student, staff, and parent manuals
  - _____ Universal, schoolwide intervention strategies
  - _____ Mission statement
  - _____ Belief system
  - _____ Goals
  - _____ Objectives
  - _____ Rules
  - _____ Routines
  - _____ Academic guidelines
  - _____ Discipline guidelines

Notes: _____

_____

_____

- *Standard subtotal* (circle one): Low ➔ High

       1   2   3   4   5

Student Support Services

- *Standard:* Counseling, social services, and health assistance are available for all students on a regular basis.
- *Indicators:* yes/no
  - _____ Career preparation
  - _____ Behavioral assessment, management, and intervention
  - _____ Guidance services
  - _____ High school diploma access
  - _____ Adult mentors
  - _____ Attendance, truancy, retention, and dropout
  - _____ ILPs (Individual Learning Plan), IEPs (Individual Education Plan), and grade point average course credit
  - _____ Transition to adult life
  - _____ Individual and group social, behavioral, and emotional counseling

Notes: _____

_____

_____

- *Standard subtotal* (circle one): Low ➔ High

       1   2   3   4   5

Equity and Diversity

- *Standard:* Physical, cultural, socioeconomic, racial, and gender differences among staff and students are considered before all program decisions are made.
- *Indicators:* yes/no
  - _____ Curriculum
  - _____ Instruction
  - _____ Assessment
  - _____ Support services (e.g., counseling, social services, and health)
  - _____ Behavior management
  - _____ Program collaboration
  - _____ Resources (e.g., materials, supplies, and equipment)

Notes: _____

_____

_____

- *Standard subtotal* (circle one): Low ➔High
  - 1   2   3   4   5

How to Monitor
Academic Performance

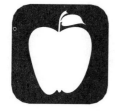 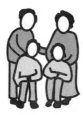 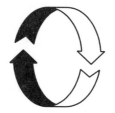  

Project Transition's unique approach is to team educators with social workers who work closely with students and their parents. The academic performance monitoring form used is shown below. The systemic approach of the program addresses areas of improving academic and interpersonal skills as well as self-esteem. In addition, it provides students with a career vocational and assessment program. Part-time jobs are provided by businesses that cooperate with the program. The program has shown an overall 55% increase in classes passed and a 63% decrease in absences. The student group has resulted in a decrease in number of suspensions and days suspended of more than 90%. Project Transition has been awarded the Crystal Star of Excellence Award by the National Dropout Prevention Center.

Academic Performance Monitoring Form

Academic Monitor Performance Form

Student _____ Date _____

Hour/ Subject	Homework Turned In	In-Class Work Done	Brought Supplies	Conduct OK	Teacher Initials
First _____					
Second _____					
Third _____					
Fourth _____					
Fifth _____					
Sixth _____					
Seventh _____					

Homework Assignments

First hour

Second hour

Third hour

Fourth hour

Fifth hour

Sixth hour

Seventh hour

Parent or Guardian Signature

How to Hire an Alternative Education Teacher

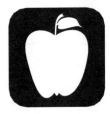 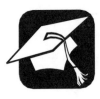  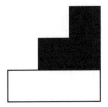

Alternative education teachers need different skills than teachers in traditional classrooms. Below is a job description that elucidates skills and qualities that one alternative education program looks for in the teachers they hire.

- ◆ Open to trying new ideas and classroom strategies
- ◆ Willing to work on a team
- ◆ Positive
- ◆ Energetic
- ◆ Willing to work on projects beyond the regular school day and school year
- ◆ Uses differentiated instruction
- ◆ Uses a variety of authentic assessment strategies
- ◆ Incorporates authentic leaning experiences in everyday lessons
- ◆ Helps students set and achieve goals
- ◆ Takes into consideration students' multiple intelligences as well as different learning styles and incorporates them into lessons
- ◆ Gives frequent feedback with students and communicates often with parents
- ◆ Provides motivational reinforcement and incentives for students
- ◆ Employs consistent yet flexible classroom discipline
- ◆ Enjoys lifelong learning and continues to take coursework to become a better teacher
- ◆ Personable and likeable
- ◆ Responsible

How to Hire an Instructional Intervention Assistant

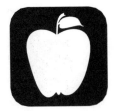  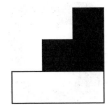

An instructional intervention assistant assists the alternative education teacher in a variety of ways. What skills should administrators look for in hiring one? Here is what one high school looks for in an instructional intervention assistant:

♦ Proactively mentors and builds positive relationships with parents and students

♦ Works with students who have been absent

♦ Makes sure students have all necessary materials

♦ Calls and/or writes to keep parents informed

♦ Circulates in class to help students, especially with group projects

♦ Troubleshoots, especially with computers

♦ Helps students stay organized

♦ Makes contacts for guest speakers

♦ Helps with field trips

♦ Takes attendance

♦ Provides one-on-one tutoring, especially math and reading

♦ Frequent feedback and interims to all students

♦ Sends classroom newsletters to parents

♦ Builds/updates Web site for teachers with assignment and lesson plans posted daily

♦ Helps students overcome daily obstacles such as turning in library books, doing make-up work, studying for and taking tests, etc.

♦ Reviews class material with students to help them prepare for tests

♦ Provides public relations, Web site, and newsletter

♦ Provides motivational reinforcement

♦ Monitors behavior

How to Monitor Student Behavior Using a Checklist

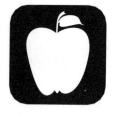 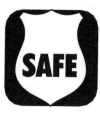 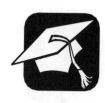 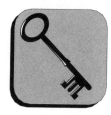 

Below is a uniform checklist of student behaviors that can be used by a variety of school personnel to monitor behaviors.

Name [   ] Grade [   ] Date [   ]

Person referring [   ]

✔ Check the appropriate response

———— School Attendance ————

☐ Change in classroom attendance

☐ In-school non-attendance

☐ Pattern of early morning tardiness

☐ Class tardiness

☐ Frequent schedule changes

☐ Class performance

———— Extracurricular Activities ————

☐ Increasing noninvolvement

☐ Not fulfilling responsibilities

☐ Loss of eligibility/dropping out

———— Behavior, Criminal/Legal ————

☐ Sells drugs/exchanges money

☐ Possesses alcohol and other drugs

- [ ] Drop in grades
- [ ] Change in class participation
- [ ] Inconsistent daily work
- [ ] Lack of motivation; apathy

- [ ] Involved in thefts and/or assaults
- [ ] Vandalizes
- [ ] Smokes
- [ ] Carries weapons

Behavior, Disruptive

- [ ] Defies rules
- [ ] Irresponsible, blames, lies
- [ ] Fights, physically abuses self and/or others
- [ ] Cheats
- [ ] Obscene language and gestures

- [ ] Has sudden outbursts, verbally abuses others
- [ ] Obtains attention in dramatic ways
- [ ] Extremely negative
- [ ] Hyperactive, nervous

Behavior, Unusual

- [ ] Talks freely about drug use
- [ ] Behaves erratically as viewed on a day-to-day basis
- [ ] Changes friends
- [ ] Hypersensitive
- [ ] Responds inappropriately
- [ ] Depressed
- [ ] Defensive
- [ ] Withdrawn, secluded, loner

- [ ] Seeks adult advice without a specific problem
- [ ] Disoriented to time
- [ ] Change in student–teacher rapport
- [ ] Attempts suicide
- [ ] Avoids contact with others
- [ ] Forgetful
- [ ] Lacks motivation
- [ ] Talks about involvement in illegal activities

Social Problems

☐ Family problems

☐ Runaway

☐ Work problems

☐ Peer problems

☐ Homeless

☐ Drinking problems

☐ Drug problems

☐ Alcohol/drug abuse

Physical Symptoms

☐ Staggers/stumbles

☐ Smells of alcohol

☐ Vomits

☐ Glassy, bloodshot eyes

☐ Physical injuries

☐ Frequent physical complaints

☐ Poor coordination

☐ Slurred speech

☐ Changes in appearance

☐ Sleepy/drowsy in class

☐ Poor hygiene

☐ Crying

Other (Please Specify)

Comments: (What behavior[s] precipitated this referral?)

Teacher/staff member's desired goal: ————————————

☐ Information only

☐ Further action requested

☐ Other (please specify) _____

_____

_____

Date received: _____

Assigned to: _____

Entering Middle and High School Student Self-Assessment

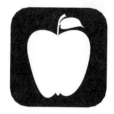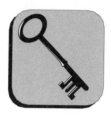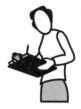

One of the best ways to get to know incoming students is to ask them to conduct a self-assessment survey. By interviewing incoming freshmen, middle and high schools can connect with students by discovering their likes, dislikes, and interests. This self-assessment was developed for an alternative program in Ohio, but it can be used by all middle and high schools.

Self-Assessment: Success Qualities You See in Yourself

Student name: _____

Enter the number that most describes you in relation to each statement:

0 = never   1 = sometimes   2 = most of the time   3 = all the time

☐ I am self-confident.

☐ I complete homework.

☐ I work independently.

☐ I get along with others.

☐ I am able to communicate ideas well.

☐ I am kind and considerate.

☐ I make good choices.

☐ I enjoy helping others.

☐ I am able to get along and work with adults.

☐ I have a positive outlook on life.

☐ I know how to gather and use information.

☐ I follow school and classroom rules.

☐ I like school.

☐ I complete class work.

☐ I am organized.

☐ I recognize the strengths of others.

☐ I express my views appropriately.

☐ I am sensitive to the needs of others.

☐ I am able to work with different kinds of people.

☐ I am a hard worker.

☐ I am even-tempered.

☐ I plan and use my time efficiently.

☐ I interact with my peers in an appropriate manner.

☐ I am a good listener.

☐ I participate in class.

My favorite subject is:

It is my favorite subject because:

I am involved in these extracurricular activities (e.g., sports, clubs, music):

I work after school (yes/no):

I work this many hours (day/night/weekend):

I spend this much time doing homework each night:

If I could change one thing about school, it would be this:

These are three of my greatest strengths:

I would like to have more of these personal skills and qualities:

After-School Experiences

Many schools provide after-school and summer enhancement programs that eliminate information loss and inspire interest in a variety of areas. Such experiences are especially important for students at risk of school failure. Tools in this module include:

"How to Create an Exemplary After-School Program" adapted from materials from The After-School Corporation (TASC), 925 Ninth Avenue, New York NY 10019 info@tascorp.org (212) 547-6950

"How to Create a High Quality After-School Program" adapted from materials from the U.S. Department of Education and the U.S. Dept. Of Justice.

"Identifying Staff Training Needs and Available Resources" adapted from materials from The After-School Corporation (TASC) 925 Ninth Avenue, New York NY 10019 info@tascorp.org (212) 547-6950

How to Create an
Exemplary After-School Program

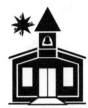 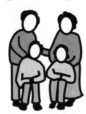 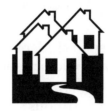 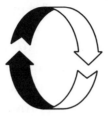 

Effective after-school programs are valuable devices for lowering the dropout rate and providing alternatives for at-risk young people. After-school programs need to focus on academic, enrichment, cultural, and recreational activities to be most effective. They also must meet the needs of the communities they serve.

The common elements of the best programs include:

♦ Collaboration between the schools and the community are key to successful programs.

♦ After-school programs need clearly defined program goals.

- Is the primary goal to raise academic achievement or provide remediation?

- Will the program include individual tutoring?

- Should the program offer enrichment such as fine or practical arts?

- Should the program offer sports or recreational activities?

- Should the major focus be on developing key skills such as study habits and test taking skills?

- Should the program offer character education, encouraging positive student behavior, and increasing students' self-esteem?

♦ A set schedule for the programs to be offered (i.e., after school, weekends, summers)

♦ Providing a safe environment during program hours.

♦ Program goals and activities linked to the school curriculum, state, and local standards.

♦ A hands-on, site-based management structure that links continuous oversight and accountability. An evaluation component, with multiple measures of success, integrated with the design allowing program planners to objectively gauge their success based on the goals set for the program.

♦ A management structure with an annual operating budget, accurate bookkeeping systems, affordable fees, and multiple funding sources.

♦ A focused program director to help ensure that the after-school program provides high quality services that meet the needs of program staff, students, families, and the community.

- Programs should hire skilled and qualified staff that are experienced in working with school-age children.
- The program should provide ongoing training for the staff.
- Volunteers who can reduce the price of the program as well as the staff-to-child ratio. The most effective staff-to-student ratio should be between 1:10.
- Programs should be safe, close to students' homes, and accessible to all who want to participate. They should have adequate space for a variety of indoor and outside activities and age-appropriate materials.
- The program should provide a nutritious snack and other meals when appropriate.
- The community and families should be involved in the program planning and be allowed to have input as to the relevancy of the program to the community as well as cultural relevancy. The program should be sensitive to the schedules and requirements of working parents and be affordable and provide transportation to and from the after-school program.

How to Create a High-Quality After-School Program

  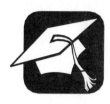  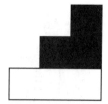

Millions of children are on their own in the morning and afternoon before and after the school bell rings. Nearly two-thirds of school-age children are in homes with working parents. Many school communities have a comprehensive system of before- and after-school care for children. The result: Millions of children are on their own, especially during the hours between 3 and 8 p.m., prime time for young people to engage in risky behavior. Statistics clearly show that rates of juvenile crime, drug use, and experimentation with tobacco, alcohol, and sex increase in the afternoon hours when many children and youth are unsupervised. A 1999 survey funded by the Charles Stewart Mott Foundation and JCPenney found that 92 percent of voters believe there should be some type of organized activity or place for children and youth to go after school every day. According to Fight Crime: Invest in Kids, the hour immediately following school dismissal yields three times as much juvenile crime as the hour before school lets out.

What Makes A High Quality After School Program?

♦ Goal setting and strong management
♦ Quality staffing
♦ Low staff/student ratios
♦ Attention to safety, health and nutrition issues
♦ Appropriate environments with adequate space and materials.
♦ Effective partnerships between parents and volunteers, schools, community-based organizations, juvenile justice agencies, law enforcement, youth-serving agencies, business leaders, community colleges, etc.
♦ Strong family involvement
♦ Coordinating learning with regular school day
♦ Links between school-day teachers and after-school staff
♦ Evaluation of program progress and effectiveness
♦ Activity choices to provide diverse educational enrichment opportunities
♦ Plans for sustainability

Identifying Staff Training Needs
and Available Resources

One of the key components of achieving success in after school programs is to train staff. Before that is done their needs must be identified as well as the resources that the program has available to fill those needs.

In 1998, The After-School Corporation (TASC) launched an initiative to improve the quantity and quality of after-school programs for students in the public schools of New York City and State. Today, the TASC After-School Program serves students in K-12 schools in more than 100 sites.

Worksheet for Identifying Staff Training Needs and Resources

Program Area	Type of Activity	Are Staff's Current Skills Sufficient?	Which Staff Need More Training?	What More Could We Do to Train Staff?	Who Could Help Us?
Sample Row:					
Academic assistance	Homework help	No	Group leaders, volunteers	• Have mentors model techniques for classroom management and use of time • Schedule bi-weekly staff meetings to discuss issues & solutions • Talk with teachers who assigned homework to better coordinate efforts • Locate research on providing homework help	• Principal • Teachers from the school day • Education specialist from our sponsoring organization • PASE ot other private vendor of staff training • Other TASC projects with strong services in this area
Academic assistance	Homework help				

Program Area	Type of Activity	Are Staff's Current Skills Sufficient?	Which Staff Need More Training?	What More Could We Do to Train Staff?	Who Could Help Us?
Academic assistance	Literacy tutoring or enrichment				
Academic assistance	Math/science tutoring or enrichment				
Academic assistance	Standardized test preparation				

Program Area	Type of Activity	Are Staff's Current Skills Sufficient?	Which Staff Need More Training?	What More Could We Do to Train Staff?	Who Could Help Us?
Academic assistance	Interdisciplinary, project-based learning				
Academic assistance	Other_____ _____ _____ _____				
Social/ emotional growth	Physical activities targeting the development of young children or adolescents				

Program Area	Type of Activity	Are Staff's Current Skills Sufficient?	Which Staff Need More Training?	What More Could We Do to Train Staff?	Who Could Help Us?
Social/emotional growth	Conflict resolution				
Social/emotional growth	Counseling for drug/alcohol abuse				
Social/emotional growth	Health services or referrals				
Social/emotional growth	Other _____ _____ _____				

Program Area	Type of Activity	Are Staff's Current Skills Sufficient?	Which Staff Need More Training?	What More Could We Do to Train Staff?	Who Could Help Us?
Youth Development	Cultural awareness activities				
Youth Development	Leadership development				
Youth Development	Problem-solving and decision making				
Youth Development	Intergenerational activities				
Youth Development	Learning through community service				
Youth Development	Other _____ _____ _____ _____				

Program Area	Type of Activity	Are Staff's Current Skills Sufficient?	Which Staff Need More Training?	What More Could We Do to Train Staff?	Who Could Help Us?
Social/ emotional growth	_____ _____ _____				
Program operations	Scheduling				
Program operations	Attendance and dismissal				
Program operations	Student grouping and seating arrangements				

Program Area	Type of Activity	Are Staff's Current Skills Sufficient?	Which Staff Need More Training?	What More Could We Do to Train Staff?	Who Could Help Us?
Program operations	Time management and classroom management				
Program operations	Interactions between students and staff				
Program operations	Partnering with the school				
Program operations	Partnering with the community				
Program operations	Other _____ _____ _____ _____				

After-School Resources

The following resources should be used to obtain additional material on after-school programs:

United States Department of Education's
   21st Century Community Learning Centers
   1-800-USA-LEARN

The David and Lucille Packard Foundation
   www.futureofchildren.org

Afterschool Alliance
   www.mott.org (type "Afterschool Alliance" in Search box)

The Finance Project
   www.financeproject.org

Children's Defense Fund
   www.childrensdefense.org

National Institute on Out-of-School Time,
   Center for Research on Women, Wellesley College
   www.niost.org

Ewing Marion Kauffman Foundation
   www.emkf.org

Council of Chief State School Officers
   www.ccsso.org

National School-Age Care Alliance
   www.nsaca.org

Local Investment Commission
   www.kclinc.org

National Governors' Association
   www.nga.org

Professional Development

Teachers who work with youth at high risk for academic failure need to feel supported and need to have an avenue by which they may continue to develop skills and techniques and learn innovative teaching strategies. Tools in this module include:

"How to Address School Problems by Prioritizing Concerns, Issues, and Tasks," developed by Dr. John V. "Dick" Hamby.

"Building Leadership Capacity Into Schools," adapted from "Hope for Urban Education," United States Department of Education, December 1999.

"How to Develop Teaming Strategies," from *Team Strategies for Success* by Dr. Mary Ann Smialek, by Mary Ann Smialek, published by Scarecrow Press, Inc., 4720 Boston Way, Lanham, Maryland 20706, 800-462-6420, used with permission.

"How to Measure The Success of Teaming Strategies," from *Team Strategies for Success* by Dr. Mary Ann Smialek, by Mary Ann Smialek, published by Scarecrow Press, Inc., 4720 Boston Way, Lanham, Maryland 20706, 800-462- 6420, used with permission.

"How to Help Students Evaluate Their Performance," adapted from material developed by Steve Berta, Manager of Student Services and Guidance at San Jose Unified School District; Howard Blonsky, San Francisco Unified School District trainer; Vicki Butler, Coordinator and Principal for special schools at the Riverside County Office of Education; Bill Deeb, Director of Research and Evaluation at Alisal Union School District; Marco Orlando, consultant with the California Department of Education; Andy Stetkevich, Staff Development Specialist for the Riverside Unified School District; used with the permission of Howard Blonsky.

"What to Look For When Observing a Student's Learning Environment," developed by Steve Berta, Manager of Student Services and Guidance at San Jose Unified School District; Howard Blonsky, San Francisco Unified School

District trainer; Vicki Butler, Coordinator and Principal for special schools at the Riverside County Office of Education Bill Deeb, Director of Research and Evaluation at Alisal Union School District; Marco Orlando, consultant with the California Department of Education; Andy Stetkevich, Staff Development Specialist for the Riverside Unified School District; used with the permission of Howard Blonsky

"How to Build the Self-Esteem of Students and Teachers," contributed by Jim Campbell, Performance Unlimited, www.performance-unlimited.com, (505) 292-8832; ©1997, used with permission.

How to Address School Problems by Prioritizing Concerns, Issues, and Tasks

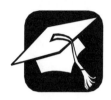

Often the staff of a school or program is faced with a number of concerns, issues, tasks, or recommendations that could be addressed when making school improvements. Given an unlimited supply of resources and time, the staff could theoretically accomplish everything it desired. However, because this is never the case in education, it is necessary to prioritize among myriad choices. The following method can be used to accomplish such prioritization:

Step 1: Write or type each concern, issue, task, recommendation, etc., on a separate note card or sheet of paper. In the upper left corner, write "Priority Level." In the upper right corner, write "Ranking."

Step 2: Study all concerns, issues, tasks, recommendations, etc., and divide them into three levels of priority as indicated below. Write the level number at the top left.

- ◆ Level 1: Items that can be addressed immediately, that cost little or nothing to address, and that are surrounded by little or no controversy
- ◆ Level 2: Items that will take a little longer to address, that have some costs related to them, and that are somewhat controversial
- ◆ Level 3: Items that will take a considerable amount of time to address, that will have considerable costs related to them, and that are controversial

The following factors, plus others you can develop, might be helpful in placing concerns, issues, tasks, or recommendations into levels. Each factor is to be rated on a five-point scale:

- ◆ Need for student improvement: rated from 1 (great need) to 5 (little need)
- ◆ Ease of implementation: rated from 1 (easy) to 5 (difficult)
- ◆ Cost in money and resources: rated from 1 (inexpensive) to 5 (expensive)
- ◆ Level of controversy: rated from 1 (little opposition) to 5 (much opposition)

Step 3: Once all items have been divided into three levels, start with the level 1 items, and prioritize each card or sheet by marking a rank in the upper right corner (1 = highest priority, 2 = second highest, etc.). When all level 1 items have been prioritized, do the same with the level 2 and level 3 items.

Step 4. When all items in each level have been ranked, begin developing a plan of action to address them. The plan should include answers to at least the following five questions:

♦ What specific outcomes are expected, what data will be collected, how will outcomes be evaluated, and how will changes be made if the action does not achieve desired outcomes?*

  * This question is listed first because people tend to overlook it or wait until the actions are completed before addressing outcomes and evaluation. Procedures for ongoing and final evaluation of actions should be determined at the beginning of a project, not at the end.

♦ What specifically will be done to achieve outcomes?

♦ Who will do it?

♦ How much will it cost, and where will resources come from?

♦ When will the task be completed?

Building Leadership Capacity Into Schools

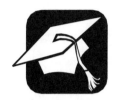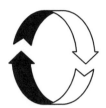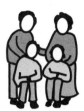

Many urban school districts experience a 50% to 70% student dropout rate. In addition, the professional life expectancy of inner city administrators is three years or fewer. The United States Department of Education issued the following improvement strategies and recommendations to urban superintendents and principals. However, they are applicable to all administrators and potential administrators.

♦ Build the capacity of principals to provide instructional leadership.

Federal, state, and local education agencies should promote strategies for building principals' capacity to provide quality instructional leadership. Strategies that build these capacities include the following:

- provide opportunities for principals to visit and learn from other schools with similar demographics that have achieved high levels of success

- assist principals in accessing, understanding, and using achievement data to guide decision-making processes

- ensure that principals have adequate time to engage in instructional support efforts on a daily basis

- give principals easy and regular access to central office personnel who can help them overcome barriers or respond constructively to problems

- give principals time for their own professional development in promising instructional practices

- mentor principals through processes for identifying, supporting, and—if necessary—firing personnel with substandard performance

♦ Channel resources in ways that provide additional instructional leadership to schools.

There is a need to develop instructional facilitator or specialist positions within schools to work with teachers on a daily basis to improve classroom instruction.

♦ Create clear, measurable, and rigorous provisions for school accountability.

Educators exhibit a deep personal sense of responsibility for improving the achievement of the children they serve. States and districts must develop policies to help frame and focus this responsibility felt by educators. States and districts need to identify ways to encourage educators to exceed minimum progress expectations and to focus on goals that exemplify quality educational services to children. It is important to realize that educators are motivated primarily by their service commitment to children, not by a need to comply with minimal district or state requirements. Effective schools go far beyond the minimum expectations of their states and districts.

♦ Ensure that accountability provisions are accompanied by adequate strategies to build capacity and provide support.

Results are most likely to come quickly if there are a few clear, consistent, measurable achievement goals and strong support from the district office to help schools achieve these goals. Accountability without capacity to succeed is only an exercise in frustration. In considering requirements for adequate yearly progress, states and districts should set ambitious requirements but also provide high levels of support. One of the most important supports is time for school personnel to engage in processes that align instruction with standards and assessments. Teachers need time to develop a deep understanding of what their students are expected to know and be able to do. Another important value of the processes comes as teachers learn that they could be a source of ideas, support, and encouragement to each other as they consider how to teach students the expected knowledge and skills.

♦ Along with accountability, provide schools with adequate flexibility, and support them in using that flexibility well.

Schools need sufficient resources to provide teachers with the materials, equipment, training, and support necessary for students to succeed. In addition, schools need the flexibility to use those resources in a manner that is tailored to the unique strengths and needs of students. Schools can then make good decisions about the use of their resources in a way that results in improved student achievement. Therefore, federal, state, and local education agencies should ensure that accountability provisions are coupled with adequate resources for schools and reasonable flexibility in the use of those resources. Also, policymakers should not assume that educators know how to use resources and decision-making opportunities well. Principals and school decision-making committees may need high-quality training that helps them use data to focus resources on critical areas of instructional need. Central office personnel can provide this support. This support can be provided through coaching associated with adoption of a comprehensive school reform model.

♦ Infuse the tenets of comprehensive school reform into all school programs.

There is a need to improve every facet of a school in a manner that will lead to the academic success of each student. Most schools do not use nationally known models of comprehensive reform.

◆ Educators need to use existing legislation, policy, and technical assistance to help them create regular opportunities for true professional development.

Professional development must be completely reconceptualized. Professionalism is developed as teachers spend time regularly planning, working, and learning with each other. Traditional notions of conferences and workshops have their place; however, they are poor substitutes for the time spent by teachers working collaboratively around instructional improvement issues.

◆ Provide resources for increasing the quantity of time made available for instruction.

After-school programs, "Saturday Schools," and extended-year programs are important vehicles for ensuring that students have opportunities to meet challenging academic standards.

◆ Strengthen legislation and provide technical assistance to encourage schools to build teachers' and parents' capacity to increase parental involvement at school.

Schools must show parents that there really is hope for their children. They need to work hard to reach out to parents and build relationships where relationships might have been poor. Current Title I legislation states that schools are required to build the capacity of parents to support the education of their children. Similarly, schools are required to build the capacity of school personnel to work effectively with parents.

◆ School districts need to better support the improvement of teaching and learning in high-poverty schools.

Research has focused largely on the school as a unit of change. Inadequate attention has been given to the role of the district in providing support to school reform efforts.

How to Develop Teaming Strategies

Schools using teamwork find greater satisfaction and higher academic success. My friend and colleague, Dr. Mary Ann Smialek, has developed several strategies to help organize teams. I am grateful to her for granting me permission to use several of her strategies.

Ten Steps to Start a New Team

Step 1: Select a project to be addressed.

Step 2: Select representative team members

Step 3: Set goals:

- Include long-term objectives (statement of purpose)
- Itemize short-term procedures (plan for completion)
- Develop a mission statement
  - Clarify focus of project
  - Set boundaries
  - Develop a schedule

Step 4: Focus on clients

- Identify clients
- Clarify clients' expectations

Step 5: Focus on work processes

- Note improvement opportunities
- Gather data
- Analyze data

Step 6: Conduct productive meetings

- Develop and use an agenda
- Employ team meeting roles
  - Facilitator
  - Timekeeper
  - Scribe (writes documentation during meeting for members)
  - Note taker (prepares minutes)
- Draft agenda for next meeting

- Summarize decisions made
- Obtain consensus on action plans
- Evaluate meeting
  - Discuss what went well
  - Note improvements that should be considered
  - Communicate meeting conclusions to others

Step 7: Carry out proposed assignments

Step 8: Document team's progress
- Choose effective methods of communication

Step 9: Initiate project closure
- Evaluate project completion
- Maintain process improvement using organizational systems and structures

Step 10: Celebrate project completion
- Recognize team efforts
- Choose appropriate ways to mark team success
  - Give small tokens of appreciation
  - Special collective breakfast, lunch, or dinner
  - Write and post positive comments
  - Provide awards or certificates
  - Give monetary compensation

How to Measure the Success of Teaming Strategies

Dr. Mary Ann Smialek has developed The Quality Empowerment Survey for Teams (QUEST), a resource designed to help teams pinpoint challenges to success and capitalize on both individual member and team strengths. QUEST clarifies and remedies areas impeding team success. In a matter of minutes, individual member and team strengths and weaknesses become evident. The team should be concerned with any team average over the team score of 2.0.

Five-Part Scale:
1 = Strongly Agree
2 = Agree
3 = Disagree
4 = Strongly disagree
5 = Undecided

Respect and Trust

_____ Team members respect me.
_____ Team members trust each other.
_____ Peers trust our team.
_____ Management respects our team.
_____ I am encouraged to take risks.

Recognition

_____ Our team recognizes my contributions.
_____ Our team expects the best from each member.
_____ Management recognizes individual efforts.
_____ Management recognizes team efforts.
_____ Our organization recognizes people for their abilities, not for who they know.

Team Communications

_____ Team members talk openly about ideas.
_____ Team members talk openly about problems.
_____ Team members actively listen to each other.
_____ Our team communicates regularly with management.

_____ Conflicts are quickly confronted and solved.

Information

_____ I have all the information needed to do my job.
_____ Our team has all the information needed to do its job.
_____ Individuals are kept informed of what is going on in the team.
_____ Individuals are kept informed of what is going on in the organization.
_____ Our team knows how to get needed information.

Decision-Making and Problem Solving

_____ Team members are encouraged to speak out.
_____ Adequate time is spent searching for innovative solutions.
_____ Team members use win-win techniques.
_____ Decisions are not evaluated without being fully discussed.
_____ Solutions are not evaluated without being fully discussed.

Resources

_____ Our team receives needed resources on time.
_____ The members of our team have all the necessary technical skills.
_____ The members of our team have all the necessary team skills.
_____ Priorities are consistently clear.
_____ Management support is readily available when needed.

Initiative and Creativity

_____ Our team has full support for taking initiative.
_____ Our team encourages individual initiative.
_____ Team initiative is encouraged by the organization.
_____ Our team easily suggests new ideas for improving processes and products.
_____ Our team easily tries new ideas for improving processes and products.

Goal Clarity

_____ Our team knows and understands the team's goals.
_____ Our team is committed to the team's goals.
_____ My individual goals match the team's goals.
_____ Our team allows me the opportunity for personal growth.
_____ Our team allows me the opportunity for career growth.

Teamwork

_____ Individuals on our team work well together to solve difficult problems.
_____ Individuals on our team focus on the team, not themselves.
_____ Our team does not focus on one or two "superstars."
_____ Our team is organized to produce a high-quality output.
_____ Our team processes are efficient and timely.

Organizational Systems and Structures

_____ Organizational policies are consistent with team goals.

_____ Our team interacts easily with other teams in our organization.

_____ Team empowerment in our organization can occur without changing major systems and structures.

_____ Our team can be empowered without changing current systems and structures.

_____ Our team can be empowered without changing current organization policies.

How to Help Students Evaluate Their Performance

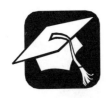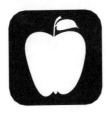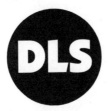

It is important that students know how to evaluate their performance in classrooms. They need to be taught what to look for an how to evaluate what they find.

Student Performance Self-Evaluation Form

Name _____ Date _____

Seldom *Sometimes* *Often* *Rate the following six items as "seldom," "sometimes," or "often."*

☐ ☐ ☐ I contributed ideas to the classroom discussion.

☐ ☐ ☐ I encouraged others as we worked.

☐ ☐ ☐ I helped give direction to the work.

☐ ☐ ☐ I followed the direction of others.

☐ ☐ ☐ I helped make decisions and solve problems.

☐ ☐ ☐ I took risks by exploring things that were new to me.

What do I contribute to the learning process? _____

_____

_____

What is the most interesting thing about what I did today?
_____

What decisions did I have to make while we were working, and how did I try to solve the problems I faced?
_____

_____

What have I learned from this particular experience, and how can I apply what I have learned to other classes and everyday life?
_____

_____

_____

What to Look for When Observing a Student's Learning Environment

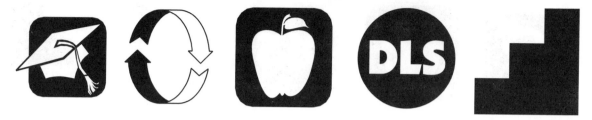

When counselors and other support personnel go into classrooms to observe students. What should they be looking for?

Student name [   ]   Date(s) [   ]

Observation within classroom

As it specifically relates to this student, indicate instructional strategies, modifications, and adaptations and their success; curricular materials used; academic and social performance; ability to work independently; verbal capabilities; motor skills; etc.

[   ]

Were any of the instructional strategies, modifications and adaptations attempted during this observation successful?

[   ]

Observations outside classroom

Comment on motor skills, social interactions, inclusion or exclusion by peers, interaction with adults, activity level, passive or aggressive behavior, etc.

[   ]

Name/title of observer [   ]

How to Build the Self-Esteem of Students and Teachers

Improving student performance is critical to improving graduation rates. A basic law in psychology states, "A person's performance will never exceed their self-esteem." Increased self-esteem of students and teachers enables both to perform at higher levels. It is not possible for one person to directly increase directly the self-esteem of another individual because only that individual can do it for himself or herself. The educational environment is ideal for implementing any or all of the following 13 behaviors by students and/or teachers that will build their own self-esteem:

- ◆ Set a goal and achieve it
- ◆ Take a risk and succeed
- ◆ Increase personal skills and abilities and apply them
- ◆ Successfully adapt to change
- ◆ Gain new knowledge and apply it
- ◆ Add value to the lives of others
- ◆ Exercise self-discipline by keeping commitments made to oneself
- ◆ Create something new
- ◆ Keep commitments made to others
- ◆ Behave congruently with personal values
- ◆ Add worth or be a positive benefit to life
- ◆ Support another person to build his or her self-esteem
- ◆ Discover a truth resulting in a "eureka" or "ah-ha" reaction

The last behavior that builds one's own self-esteem produces a win-win situation for both teachers and students. Teachers automatically increase their own self-esteem as they support their peers and their students in building self-esteem. Similarly, students expand their own self-esteem as they support their peers in doing the same. Behaviors that provide such support are as follows:

- ◆ Validate another person as a worthwhile human being at every opportunity to do so
- ◆ Create an environment that enables that person to experience any of the above behaviors that build self-esteem
- ◆ Privately reinforce the other person for minor success with any of the above behaviors that build self-esteem

Publicly acknowledge the other person for major success with any of the above behaviors that build self-esteem.

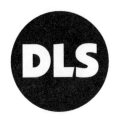

Diverse Learning Styles and Multiple Intelligences

When educators show students that there are different ways to learn, students find new and creative ways to solve problems, achieve success, and become lifelong learners. Tools in this module include:

"How to Define the Eight Multiple Intelligences," adapted from *Pondering Learning: Connecting Multiple Intelligences and Service Learning*, Corporation for National Service and the National Dropout Prevention Center at Clemson University. Used with permission.

"How to Link Multiple Intelligences with Careers," developed By Franklin P. Schargel.

"How to Use Mediated Learning Experiences and Instrumental Enrichment in the Classroom," contributed by Linda Borsum, Quality Learning Systems International, 4950 West Dickman Road, Suite B-3, Battle Creek, Michigan 49015, 800-379-2322, www.qlsi.com, used with permission.

How to Define the Eight Multiple Intelligences

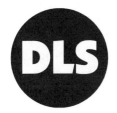 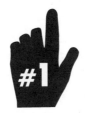 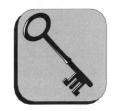 

Dr. Howard Gardner introduced his Multiple Intelligence theory in *Frames of Mind* (1983). Dr. Gardner believes that people are smart in different ways. Although Dr. Gardner introduced eight *separate* intelligences, they are rarely expressed separately. People are complex creatures with overlapping intelligences, with some intelligences being stronger than others. The figures on pages 98 and 99 the descriptions of the eight intelligences combines occupations with the eight intelligences. Ask students to match their intelligences with the occupations listed.

♦ **Verbal and Linguistic Intelligence (Word Smart)**

People with this intelligence can often communicate effectively through speaking and writing, and they are typically strong readers and listeners as well as debaters. They may have a passion for poetry, humor, storytelling, debating, creative writing, and the like.

♦ **Logical and Mathematical Intelligence (Logic Smart)**

This intelligence is associated with what we call "scientific thinking" and mathematical reasoning, including the forming and testing of hypotheses, deductive and inductive thinking, manipulating numbers, and recognizing abstract patterns. Such people are good at figuring things out, analyzing things, and solving problems in subjects such as math and science.

♦ **Intrapersonal Intelligence (Self Smart)**

Intrapersonal intelligence involves a deep sense of understanding oneself, one's strengths and weaknesses, one's feelings; it includes the capacity to be self-reflective. People with this intelligence are good at setting goals, mediating, assessing situations, and monitoring their own thinking.

♦ **Interpersonal Intelligence (People Smart)**

Interpersonal intelligence is characterized by the capacity to understand others and the fine nuances of their moods, feelings, body language, and motivations. It also includes a strong capacity to communicate both verbally and nonverbally with others in both groups and one on one. People with this intelligence are also good at sharing their opinions and demonstrate a heightened sense of understanding the personalities and feelings of others.

+ **Visual and Spatial Intelligence (Picture Smart)**

Visual and spatial intelligence involves the ability to create internal mental pictures and to comprehend the visual world. People highly developed in this intelligence are good at creating pictures in their mind whether it is by illustrating those images (as in the case of an artist) or mentally conceptualizing the images (as in the case of an interior designer). Such people demonstrate the intellectual capacity of seeing beyond two-dimensional limitations. They are also sensitive to colors, shapes, lines, and images. They may like to draw, paint, sculpt, design, and/or visualize and imagine things.

+ **Musical and Rhythmic Intelligence (Music Smart)**

People who are strong in musical and rhythmic intelligence may be musical themselves or keen listeners who are appreciative of fine music. Such people enjoy things such as singing, playing musical instruments, beating drums, humming, writing songs, and performing.

+ **Bodily and Kinesthetic Intelligence (Body Smart)**

Bodily and kinesthetic intelligence includes the ability to use the body to express emotion and to have grace and control of motion in areas such as dance and sports. People strong in this intelligence learn well by doing. They are often gifted with their hands and skilled at building and inventing.

+ **Naturalist Intelligence (Nature Smart)**

Naturalist intelligence refers to the ability to recognize patterns and classify plants, animals, minerals, and other parts of the natural environment such as clouds or rocks. They are good at analyzing data from nature. They often like hiking, camping, fishing, digging for fossils, or other activities related to the natural environment.

How to Link Multiple Intelligences with Careers

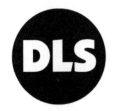 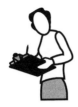   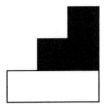

Dr. Howard Gardner introduced his Multiple Intelligence theory in Frames of Mind (1983). Dr. Gardner believes that people are smart in different ways. The following charts combine occupations with the eight intelligences. Teachers should ask students match their occupational preferences with the intelligence that dominates that field.

Blank Occupations and Intelligences Chart

Occupation/Job	Naturalist (Nature Smart)	Verbal/Linguistic (Word Smart)	Interpersonal (People Smart)	Logical/Mathematical (Logic Smart)	Intrapersonal (Self Smart)	Visual/Spatial (Picture Smart)	Bodily/Kinesthetic (Body Smart)	Musical/Rhythmic (Music Smart)
Accountant								
Actor/Actress								
Athlete								
Botanist								
Builder								
Comedian								
Computer Programmer								
Dancer								
Gardener								
Interior Designer								
Journalist								
Lawyer								
Mathematician								
Musician								
Photographer								
Pilot								
Poet								
Politician								
Sculptor								
Sound Engineer								
Surgeon								
Teacher								
Therapist								
Translator								
Typist								
Writer								

Completed Occupations and Intelligences Chart.

Occupation/Job	Naturalist (Nature Smart)	Verbal/Linguistic (Word Smart)	Logical/Mathematical (Logic Smart)	Interpersonal (People Smart)	Intrapersonal (Self Smart)	Visual/Spatial (Picture Smart)	Bodily/Kinesthetic (Body Smart)	Musical/Rhythmic (Music Smart)
Accountant			✓					
Actor/Actress							✓	
Athlete							✓	
Botanist	✓							
Builder							✓	
Comedian		✓						✓
Computer Programmer								
Dancer						✓	✓	
Gardener	✓							
Interior Designer					✓	✓		
Journalist					✓			
Lawyer		✓			✓			
Mathematician			✓					
Musician								✓
Photographer						✓		
Pilot						✓		
Poet		✓						
Politician				✓	✓			
Sculptor						✓		
Sound Engineer								✓
Surgeon								
Teacher				✓				
Therapist				✓				
Translator		✓			✓			
Typist		✓					✓	
Writer		✓						

How to Use Mediated Learning Experiences and Instrumental Enrichment in the Classroom

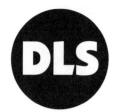  

Professor Reuven Feuerstein is a cognitive psychologist who rejected the idea that intelligence is fixed. He developed a program to build the cognitive functions of at-risk youth. Feuerstein's Instrumental Enrichment (FIE) program established the principle that all individuals can learn. FIE is today taught in more than 29 languages and in 33 counties. Mediated learning experience is a process designed to help the student by doing the following:

- ♦ Encouraging autonomous learning
- ♦ Unlocking a student's potential
- ♦ Promoting the use of effective thinking skills
- ♦ Developing interaction skills
- ♦ Improving effective parenting
- ♦ Remediating cognitive dysfunctions
- ♦ Analyzing students' cognitive strengths and weaknesses
- ♦ Encouraging metacognition, i.e., "thinking about thinking"

The first of the following two exercises is directed at students (learners). In the second, Feuerstein directs teachers to complete a classroom checklist.

Exercise One: Fuerstein's Cognitive Functions

- ♦ Gathering all the information you need (input)
  - Using your senses (listening, seeing, smelling, tasting, touching, feeling) to gather clear and complete information (clear perception)
  - Using a system or plan so that you do not skip or miss something important or repeat yourself (systematic exploration)
  - Giving the thing you gather through your senses and your experience a name so that you can remember it more clearly and talk about it (labeling)
  - Describing things and events in terms of where and when they occur (temporal and spatial referents)
  - Deciding on the characteristics of a thing or event that always stay the same, even when changes take place (conservation, constancy, and object permanence)

- Organizing the information you gather by considering more than one thing at a time (using two sources of information)
- Being precise and accurate when it matters (need for precision)

◆ Using the information we have gathered (elaboration)
- Defining what the problem is, what you are being asked to do, and what you must figure out (analyzing disequilibrium)
- Using only that part of the information you have gathered that is relevant (i.e., that applies to the problem) and ignoring the rest (relevance)
- Having a good picture in your mind of what you are looking for or what you must do (interiorization)
- Making a plan that will include the steps you need to take to reach your goal (planned behavior)
- Remembering and keeping in mind the various pieces of information you need (broadening our mental field)
- Looking for the relationship by which separate objects, events, and experiences can be tied together (projecting relationships)
- Comparing objects and experiences to others to see what is similar and what is different (comparative behavior)
- Finding the class or set to which the new object or experience belongs (categorization)
- Thinking about different possibilities and figuring out what would happen if you were to choose one or another (hypothetical thinking)
- Using logic to prove things and defend your opinion (logical evidence)

◆ Expressing the solution to the problem (output)
- Being clear and precise in your language to be sure that there is no question as to what your answer is; putting yourself into the "shoes" of the listener to be sure that your answer will be understood (overcoming egocentric communication)
- Thinking things through before you answer instead of immediately trying to answer and making a mistake and then trying again (overcoming trial-and-error)
- Counting to ten (at least!) so that you do not say or do something you will be sorry for later (restraining impulsive behavior)
- Not fretting or panicking if you cannot answer a question for some reason even though you "know" the answer; leaving the question for a little while and then, when returning to it, using a strategy to help you find the answer (overcoming blocking)

Exercise Two: Mediated Learning Experience in the Classroom

◆ Teaching style
- I have made sure the atmosphere favors communication.
- I have prepared the material needed to perform planned activities.
- I have explicitly stated the goals of the activity and the way I plan to follow up.

- I have aroused interest and curiosity using different strategies.
- I have presented the topic using more than one operating tool.
- After assigning the task, I have checked the student's understanding of my instructions.
- My explanation was followed by some practice on the student's part.
- When needed, I have illustrated the topic repeatedly and in different ways.
- I have devoted the last part of the lesson to summarizing and consolidating previously acquired elements.
- I have provided extra material.
- Today I worked on _____.
- Tomorrow I will work on _____.

♦ Development of cognitive functions
- I have checked on previously acquired knowledge in relation to new topics.
- I have reminded students of previous experiences and/or tasks to enhance connections.
- I have increased the level of complexity step by step.
- I have introduced the same term, concept, strategy, and modality in different situations to stress its applicability across different domains.
- I have developed in students an awareness and understanding of their own thinking process.
- I have created situations in which students are asked to think rather than re-produce information.
- I have presented the topic relying chiefly on an inductive approach.
- I have put little emphasis on extrinsic motivation (marks, competition, not be-ing reproached).
- I have favored intrinsic motivation by making the task attractive.
- I have used mistakes to change my procedure and ease students' understand-ing of class material.
- Today I worked on _____.
- Tomorrow I will work on _____.

♦ Teacher as mediator
- I have compiled the behaviors I expect of my students (i.e., being on time, timely delivery of work, willing to accept suggestions, etc.).
- I have showed discouragement when faced with failure.
- I have changed my behavior and attitude in relation to class response to a spe-cific contest.
- I have employed self-correction and used mistakes as resources to find more appropriate ways to teach.
- I have planned tools and occasions for self-evaluation.
- I have contributed examples from my own life experiences.
- I have explicitly stated the values in relation to the task.
- I have emphasized the goals and possible use of specific subject matter.

- I have organized activities that may establish a link between the class and the outer environment and adult patterns of behavior.
- I have disseminated the results of class activities.
- Today I worked on _____.
- Tomorrow I will work on _____.

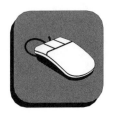

Instructional Technologies

Technology offers some of the best opportunities for delivering instruction that engages students in authentic learning, addresses multiple intelligences, and adapts to students' learning styles. Tools in this module include:

"What Are the Questions Schools Need to Answer About Using Technology?," adapted from "An Educator's Guide to Evaluating the Use of Technology in Schools and Classrooms," United States Department of Education, Office of Educational Research and Improvement, published 1988.

"Rubrics for Measuring Technological Competencies," developed by the Utah Technology Awareness Project, permission to use granted by Corey Stokes, 800-836-4396, www.uen.org/cgi-bin/websql/utahlink.

What Are the Questions Schools Need to Answer About Using Technology?

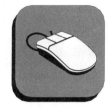 

The use of technology has many advantages, as well as disadvantages, for school use. Dynamic technological improvements in instruction must be balanced against the high costs and rapid obsolescence. What do schools need to know before deciding whether to use technology?

- Are teachers using technology in their instruction?
- Are teachers using technology effectively in their instruction?
- Is technology positively affecting student work and motivation?
- Is technology improving student work and standardized test scores?
- Are teachers and other staff members receiving adequate training in the use of technology?
- Who is evaluating software? Is the use of technology alleviating some of the school's problems?
- Is the use of computers more cost-effective than other options? How does the school and the school district use professional development activities to get the most value for the money that is to be, or has been, spent?
- Will the use of computers provide students with job opportunities in the future?
- Has adequate funding been provided to update, repair, and secure the machines?
- Will *all* teachers have the training they need to help students learn how to use computers and the Internet?
- What will have to be measured to show that there has been significant student improvement?
- Has the technology been integrated into the curriculum? Or is it being treated as an appendage to existing curriculum?

Rubrics for Measuring Technological Competencies

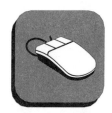 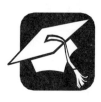 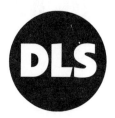 

As society and the workplace become more compute dependent, all students will need to be technologically prepared. How should schools measure the competency of those who use computers and software? The state of Utah has developed a series of rubrics to measure the effectiveness of computer use.

Basic Concepts and Skills

Each subcategory has four stages of awareness that are described as follows: 1 = early, 2 = emergent, 3 = fluent, and 4 = proficient.

- ◆ **Subcategory:** *Mousing Skills*

    1. Knows that mouse movement correlates with pointer movement on the screen and is used for interacting with objects on the screen.

    2. Can point, press, click and drag, and double-click with the mouse. Can apply mouse movement skills to touch pad, track balls, laptop-eraser mouse, and joysticks. Recognizes when the computer has registered a mouse click. Recognizes that there are different uses for each mouse button (left/right or primary/secondary.)

    3. Knows how to shift-click to select and deselect multiple items. Knows how to create and use a selection rectangle for multiple selections. Know the different functions of a single-click and a double-click and knows when it is appropriate to use each type of click. If using a two-button mouse, can change the primary and secondary buttons. Knows when and where it is appropriate to use the primary and secondary mouse buttons.

    4. Fast, smooth mouse movement across the screen. Make few wrong turns, and rarely grabs the wrong screen object. Accomplishes movement across the screen in short time. Uses modifier keys to select multiple icons and items. Knows keyboard shortcuts to mouse actions. Can adjust mouse settings in the control panel.

- ◆ **Subcategory:** *Graphic User Interface Skills*

    1. Knows how to pull down a menu. Knows how to click a radio button in a dialog box. Can scroll with at least one method. Can open and close a window or a folder. Can launch programs using the Windows start button or pull-down menu.

    2. Knows that scrolling can be done both horizontally and vertically. Can drag windows from one screen location to another. Can resize, minimize, and

maximize windows. Understands and can scroll with the scroll bar using different scrolling methods.

3. Can tile and arrange icons. Can identify different types of icons. Can rename icons. Can switch between windows of different applications. Knows how to "click" a button without the mouse. Can use pop-up menus.

4. Can adjust appearance of the desktop (e.g., fonts, colors, and backgrounds). Can use the command keys to choose actions. Can create short cuts or aliases. Can customize palettes such as the Launcher. Can change views in windows.

♦ **Subcategory:** *File Management and Operating System*

1. Knows how to insert and eject a floppy disk, CD, and DVD. Can save a file from both inside applications and outside applications in the finder or file manager. Can keep disks physically safe. Can select, copy, and paste text and graphics. Understands the difference between closing, minimizing, and hiding windows and quitting a program.

2. Knows where a saved file was saved. Knows the most appropriate place to save a file (i.e., floppy, hard drive, network drive). Can format and initialize a disk. Knows how to insert and eject CD-ROMs. Knows how to write-protect a floppy disk. Knows how to give a file a unique name while saving. Knows how to "find." Can back up documents. Can copy and paste between documents from different applications.

3. Works comfortably in at least one operating system. Knows how to locate and use control panels. Understands the directory tree of multiple disks. Knows how to change the name of an existing file. Knows how to duplicate files in the same directory tree. Knows how to organize the directory tree for efficiency. Knows how to monitor the space remaining on a drive. Can save a file as a different file type such as saving a Word Perfect document as a plain ASCII text.

4. Can work comfortably in more than one operating system. Aware of the location of most files on local operating system. Deletes unnecessary files from the computer when appropriate. Knows how to back up data and has a systematic plan in place to back up files regularly. Knows how to restore files from a back up. Understands file attributes and the differences between file types, including application-specific documents, applications, and system file. Understand RAM allocation of applications and how to troubleshoot for low RAM conditions. Understands the difference between hard drive storage capacity and RAM. Can set up a start-up folder.

♦ **Subcategory:** *Setup and Basic Troubleshooting*

1. Can power up a computer. Knows how to check computer, monitor, power strip, and wall outlet for power connections. Can shut down the computer appropriately. Writes down error messages to report problems.

2. Can perform a soft reboot of the operating systems with keystrokes. Can set an operating system such as a Windows '98 or Macintosh 10X computer. Can troubleshoot basic things before contacting the technology specialist, e.g., power to machine and monitor, plugs, and power buttons; floppy disk without system file is ejected. Aware of basic computer care issues such as routine cleaning, static protection, temperature control, and physical placement.

3. Regularly uses routine maintenance utilities such as defragmenter, scan disk, or rebuilding the desktop. Knows the typical symptoms of software problems including virus-provoked anomalies, corrupted preferences files, misplaced system files, system software conflicts, and orphaned shortcuts or aliases. Knows how to tell if the network is available to a computer. Knows to check that a network cable is connected to the computer. Can install stand-alone application software. Knows how to find out how much RAM and hard drive storage space a computer has. Has access to and use a virus checker. Can express problems clearly to a technology specialist.

4. Can reconfigure and troubleshoot the network software. Can run disk utility software to diagnose a software problem. Has access to, uses, and regularly updates a virus checker. Knows how to swap hardware devices to check or problems and can recognize when the problem is faulty hardware. Knows when it is time to call a technology specialist. Can connect a projection device such as a TV, LCD panel, or LCD projector to a computer. Can install new hardware such as a modem, Ethernet card, or speakers.

♦ **Subcategory:** *Printing Skills*

1. Can determine if a machine has a printer and cable attached. Can load paper. Can use software to select a printer.

2. Can change toner or ribbon and can clear paper jams. Understands how to change default printer. Can change print parameters such as numbers of copies, paper orientation, margins, proportions, etc. Can troubleshoot local printer problems.

3. Can troubleshoot a network printer job. Understands what a print spool does and how to manage it with software. Can install a print driver. Can add a new printer to a local computer.

4. Can set up and manage a network print queue.

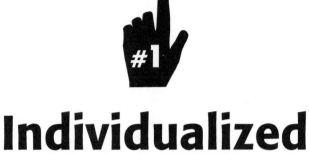

Individualized Instruction

A customized individual learning program for each student allows teachers to be flexible with the instructional program and extracurricular activities. The tool in this module is:

"How to Develop Individual Learning Plans," Chugash School District, Richard DeLorenzo, Superintendent; Debbie Treece, Quality Schools Coordinator; and superb staff. Chugash School District, 9312 Vanguard Drive, No.100 Anchorage, Alaska 99507, 704-907-7400, www.chugashschools.com, used with permission.

How to Develop
Individual Learning Plans

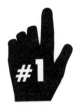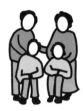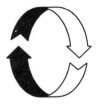

"One-size fits all" instruction doesn't work. It never did! We are aware that children learn in different ways and in different time frames. Although it is difficult for those people who mastered the system to comprehend that concept, the reality is that learning must be tailored to the individual needs of the student. This is a major challenge, in terms of time, and systems or schools that can provide educators with the time to design, develop, interview, and complete an individualized learning plan will find it really worthwhile. The plans below focus on the strengths and areas of student improvement. If individual educacion plans (IEPs) work for special education students, then individual learning plans (ILS; pages 114 through 120) will work for both at-risk and all other students.

The district is located in Anchorage, Alaska, but it draws students from 22,000 square miles of mostly isolated and rural areas of south central Alaska. The Chugash school system occupies a unique place in American education. This small school district (214 students) is among the first winners of the Malcolm Baldrige National Quality Award in Education. With 30 faculty and staff members, Chugash is the smallest organization to ever win a Baldrige Award. This means it has been recognized as the finest school district in America. More important, the district has raised its test scores significantly and lowered its dropout rate of extremely high at-risk students.

The staff, teachers, and administrators credit the development and use of ILPs as a resource that helped the district surpass the rest of Alaska's schools' average in high school graduation–qualifying (HSGQ) scores in all three subject areas of reading, writing, and math in all four grades tested. In addition, the percentage of Chugash tenth-graders who passed the HSGQ ranked first in writing, third in math, and seventeenth in reading among the state's 54 districts.

Example of ILP

Individual Learning Plan

Student [_____]   Date [_____]

Present Level of Performance

	Student	Teacher
Testing Data	[_____]	[_____]
Weaknesses	[_____]	[_____]
Goals	[_____]	[_____]

Goals/Objectives	Steps for Success	Evaluation
Standard Area Targets Addressed	What will I do to accomplish this?	How will I prove I have learned this?

Student Signature/Parent Signature [_____]   [_____]

Teacher Signature/Aide Signature [_____]   [_____]

Chugach School District ILP Standards Continuum

Personal Awareness

PS 1.1   Understands what it means to be a good student

PS 2.2   Defines and demonstrates respect for self, others, and property

PS 3.1   Identifies personal strengths and weaknesses

PS 4.7   Shares personal awareness of values and recognizes strengths and weaknesses

PS 5.5   Demonstrates personal awareness through sharing of values, interests, strengths, and weaknesses

PS 6.5   Displays personal responsibility (time management, scheduling, problem solving, budgeting, decision making, etc.) [partial standard]

PS 7.3   Evaluates responsibility and consequences of choices and actions

PS 8.4   Strives for personal growth through commitment to lifelong learning

Goal Setting

PS 2.3   Understands the importance of setting goals

PS 3.3   Exhibits self-discipline [partial standard]

PS 3.4   Practices decision making [partial standard]

PS 3.5   Practices a goal-setting process to establish short-term and long-term goals

PS 5.3   Demonstrates commitment to learning and personal development (ILP, life skills portfolio)

PS 6.5   Displays personal responsibility (time management, scheduling, problem solving, budgeting, decision making, etc.) [partial standard]

PS 7.3   Evaluates responsibility and consequences of choices and actions

PS 8.2   Makes informed decisions after exploring options and weighing consequences

PS 8.4   Strives for personal growth through commitment to lifelong learning

Steps for Success and assessment: Problem Solving and Decision Making

PS 3.3   Exhibits self-discipline and pride in work [partial standard]

PS 3.4   Practices decision making, conflict resolution, and problem solving strategies

PS 3.5   Practices a goal setting process to establish short-term and long-term goals

PS 4.5   Applies problem-solving skills and good study skills

PS 5.2   Applies conflict resolution and critical thinking skills to a variety of situations

PS 5.3   Demonstrates commitment to learning and personal development (ILP, life skills portfolio)

PS 5.4   Develops a strong personal ethic (quality task completion, best effort, and honesty) [partial standard]

PS 6.2   Makes deadlines [partial standard]

PS 6.5   Displays personal responsibility (time management, scheduling, problem solving, budgeting, decisions making, etc.) [partial standard]

PS 7.1   Demonstrates ability to find community or continuing education resources (health clinics, city and tribal councils, employment services, trade school, college, etc.)

PS 7.3   Evaluates responsibility and consequences of one's choices and actions

PS 8.2   Makes informed decisions after exploring options and weighing consequences

PS 8.4   Strives for personal growth through commitment to lifelong learning

PS 8.5   Proposes strategies and support structures to assist in dealing with problems associated with family, school, and work

Chugach School District middle-level ILP scoring guide: Personal development levels 3, 4, and 5

	−*Emerging*	✓*Developing*	✦*Proficient*	✷*Advanced*
Personal Awareness (Values and Strengths and Weaknesses)	• 3.1 Unwilling to participate and/or demonstrates inappropriate behavior • 4.7 Expresses difficulty when assessing own values, strengths, and weaknesses • 5.5 Does not demonstrate personal awareness by sharing values, strengths, and weaknesses	• 3.1 Strengths and weaknesses that are not identified may stand out to others • 4.7 Begins to assessment own values, interests, strengths, and weaknesses • 5.5 Begins to demonstrate personal awareness by sharing values, and strengths and weaknesses	• 3.1 Identifies at least three strengths and weaknesses • 4.7 Shares values and recognizes at least three strengths and weaknesses • 5.5 Demonstrates personal awareness by sharing values, and strengths, and weaknesses	• 3.1 Identifies more than three strengths and weaknesses and/or identifies values • 4.7 Begins to analyze values, interests, strengths, and weaknesses to set goals • 5.5 Analyzes values, interests, strengths, and weaknesses effectively to set goals
Goal Setting	• 3.3, 3.4, 3.5 Shows little understanding of importance of goal setting; teacher must identify goal • 5.3 Goal shows no commitment to learning and personal development	• 3.3, 3.4, 3.5 Understands the importance of setting goals; begins to self-direct goal setting process • 5.3 Goal is chosen without much consideration of commitment to learning	• 3.3, 3.4, 3.5 Goal reflects student interest and shows the ability to use a goal-setting process • 5.3 Goal clearly reflects a commitment to learning and personal development and is aligned with the report card	• 3.3, 3.4, 3.5 Goal shows reflection of strengths and weaknesses • 5.3 Exhibits self-direction and self-motivation in the ILP

| Steps for Success: Problem Solving and Decision Making | • 3.3, 3.4, 3.5 Unwilling to show effort to complete steps and/or demonstrates inappropriate behavior

• 4.5 Steps demonstrate little understanding of the goal-setting process and display limited problem-solving skills and/or good study skills

• 5.2, 5.3, 5.4 Steps reflect limited critical thinking skills and personal ethics (e.g., quality task completion, best effort) | • 3.3, 3.4, 3.5 Steps show a lack of self-discipline and/or application of problem-solving skills

• 4.5 Steps show a lack of problem-solving skills and/or good study skills

• 5.2, 5.3, 5.4 Steps reflect some understanding of commitment to learning and personal development and may show a need for critical thinking skills and personal ethics (e.g., quality task completion, best effort) | • 3.3, 3.4, 3.5 Steps show self-discipline and problem-solving strategies (effort is made to complete steps independently)

• 4.5 Steps are partially self-directed and may show the use of problem-solving skills and/or good study skills that may be applied when completing steps or when in need of teacher guidance (student self-directs other studies when the teacher is helping others)

• 5.2, 5.3, 5.4 Steps clearly reflect a commitment to learning and personal development through some mastery of steps for success that are self-directed and show critical thinking skills and personal ethics (e.g., quality task completion, best effort) | • 3.3, 3.4, 3.5 Steps are partially mastered with self-direction

• 4.5 Steps are partially mastered with self-direction, and student may encourage others to use problem-solving skills and/or good study skills through modeling, leading, and coaching

• 5.2, 5.3, 5.4 Steps for success are mastered with self-direction and may enrich learning beyond identified goal |

Assessment (Problem Solving and Decision Making)	• 3.3, 3.4, 3.5 Limited effort to complete assessment and/or shows inappropriate behavior • 4.5 Displays limited problem-solving skills and/or good study skills • 5.2, 5.3, 5.4 Shows limited critical thinking skills and/or effort to make decisions about assessment	• 3.3, 3.4, 3.5 With teacher prompting, considers assessment with teacher guidance • 4.5 Begins to use problem-solving to consider assessment that relates to goal • 5.2, 5.3, 5.4 Begins to use critical thinking skills to make decisions about assessment	• 3.3, 3.4, 3.5 Uses decision-making skills to consider assessment without teacher guidance • 4.5 Uses problem-solving and decision-making skills to consider assessment that clearly relates to goal • 5.2, 5.3, 5.4 Independently aligns assessment to goal and demonstrates good critical thinking skills	• 3.3, 3.4, 3.5 Uses decision-making skills to consider assessment that clearly relates to goal • 4.5 Independently aligns and/or creates assessment to goal by using problem-solving and decision-making skills • 5.2, 5.3, 5.4 Displays excellent critical thinking skills that leads to student-created assessment and self-direction in personal development

Personal Awareness

PS 3.1   Identifies personal strengths and weaknesses

PS 4.7   Shares personal awareness of values and recognizes strengths and weaknesses

PS 5.5   Demonstrates personal awareness through sharing of values, interests, strengths, and weaknesses

Goal Setting

PS 3.3   Exhibits self-discipline [partial standard]

PS 3.4   Practices decision-making [partial standard]

PS 3.5   Practices a goal-setting process to establish short-term and long-term goals

PS 5.3   Demonstrates commitment to learning and personal development (ILP, life skills portfolio)

Steps for Success and Assessment: Problem-Solving and Decision-Making

PS 3.3   Exhibits self-discipline and pride in work [partial standard]

PS 3.4   Practices decision-making, conflict resolution, and problem-solving strategies

PS 3.5   Practices a goal-setting process to establish short-term and long-term goals

PS 4.5   Applies problem-solving skills and good study skills

PS 5.2   Applies conflict resolution and critical thinking skills to a variety of situations

PS 5.3   Demonstrates commitment to learning and personal development (ILP, life skills portfolio)

PS 5.4   Develops a strong personal ethic (quality task completion, best effort, and honesty) [partial standard]

Chugach School District upper-level ILP scoring guide: Personal development levels 6, 7, and 8

	−*Emerging*	✓*Developing*	✦*Proficient*	✱*Advanced*
Personal Awareness (Values, Strengths, and Weaknesses): Overall ILP	• 6.5 ILP does not reflect personal awareness • 7.3 ILP demonstrates personal awareness but does not reflect evaluation of responsibility • 8.4 Able to evaluate responsibility of personal awareness but has limited plans and strategies to address strengths and weaknesses	• 6.5 Demonstrates personal awareness, but ILP does not reflect responsibility of awareness • 7.3 Begins to evaluate responsibility of personal awareness through the ILP • 8.4 Evaluates responsibility of personal awareness and begins to plan strategies to address strengths and weaknesses	• 6.5 Displays personal responsibility through identifying values, strengths, and weaknesses and addressing them in the ILP through the use of the report card • 7.3 Evaluation of the following is evident in the ILP: responsibility of personal awareness; consequences of choices and actions; alignment of goals, steps, and assessment to the report card • 8.4 A commitment to personal growth and life-long learning is evident in the ILP through planning strategies that build on strengths and address weaknesses from evaluation of personal awareness	• 6.5 Effectively plans to improve upon strengths and weaknesses through ILP and the report card • 7.3 Report card is used to independently align ILP goals, steps, and assessments that build on strengths and addresses weaknesses • 8.4 Report card is used to independently align ILP goals, steps, and assessments that build on strengths and addresses weaknesses

Goal Setting	• 6.5 Goal is limited in it reflection of personal responsibility	• 6.5 Goal partially reflects personal responsibility and is aligned with the report card	• 6.5 Goal reflects personal responsibility and is aligned with the report card	• 6.5 Goal reflects weaknesses and/or levels on the report card that are low
	• 7.3 Goal is limited in its reflection of an evaluation of personal responsibility	• 7.3 Goal is aligned to the report card and partially reflects an evaluation of personal responsibility	• 7.3 Goal reflects an evaluation of responsibility and the consequences of choices and actions and is aligned with the report card	• 7.3 Goal reflects weaknesses and/or levels on the report card that are low
	• 8.2 Goal is limited in reflection of an informed decision	• 8.2 Goal partially reflects an informed decision	• 8.2 Goal reflects an informed decision that explores options and weighs consequences and is aligned with the report card	• 8.2 Goal integrates multiple standards

Steps for Success: Problem Solving and Decision Making	• 6.5 Partially self-directed steps are limited in at least one of the following areas: decision making and problem solving skills, time management, or scheduling	• 6.5 Self-directed steps show decision-making and problem-solving skills but may need more direction in time management and scheduling	• 6.5 Self-directed steps show decision-making and problem-solving skills, time management (6.2 makes deadlines), and scheduling	• 6.5 All steps are organized into a schedule, assigned deadlines (6.2), and aligned with goal and assessment
	• 7.3 Self-directed steps are limited in the reflection of an evaluation of responsibility, choices, and actions	• 7.3 Self-directed steps begin to demonstrate an evaluation of responsibility and consequences of choices and actions	• 7.3 Self-directed steps demonstrate evaluation of responsibility and consequences of choices and actions and /or (7.1) the ability to find community and continuing education resources that assist in reaching goal	• 7.1 , 7.3 All steps have resources identified, and some are aligned to standards and district-mandated assessments
	• 8.2, 8.4 Self-directed steps demonstrate an evaluation of responsibility but are limited in the following areas: exploring options, making informed decisions, and weighing consequences	• 8.2, 8.4 Self-directed steps reflect a commitment to personal growth but do not demonstrate one or more of the following: exploring options, making informed decisions, or weighing consequences	• 8.2, 8.4 Self-directed steps reflect a commitment to personal growth and demonstrate exploring options, making informed decisions, weighing consequences, and (optional 8.5) proposing strategies to assist with problems in the family, school, and work	• 8.2, 8.4 Alternative steps have been explored, identified, and planned
				• 8.5 Steps reflect strategies to assist with problems in the family, school, and work and have been aligned to assessment and movement on the report card

Assessment: Problem Solving and Decision Making	• 6.5 Limited use of problem-solving and decision-making skills to partially create, align, and adapt assessment • 7.3 Creates, aligns, and adapts assessment that is limited in reflection of evaluation of responsibility • 8.2, 8.4 Creates, aligns, and adapts assessment but shows limited demonstration of 1, 2, 3➜	• 6.5 Uses problem-solving and decision-making skills to partially create, align, and adapt assessment or align mandated assessment • 7.3 Creates, aligns, and adapts assessment that partially reflects an evaluation of responsibility • 8.2, 8.4 Creates, aligns, and adapts assessment and begins to demonstrate 1, 2, 3➜	• 6.5 Uses problem-solving and decision-making skills to create, align, and adapt assessment or aligns mandated assessment • 7.3 Creates, aligns, and adapts assessment or aligns mandated assessment that reflects evaluation of responsibility • 8.2, 8.4 Independently created, aligned, or adapted assessment clearly reflects commitment to personal growth and demonstrates exploring options, making informed decisions, and weighing consequences	• 6.2 Assessments are identified for each step • 7.3 Multitype assessments are identified for each step • 8.2, 8.4 Multitype assessments are identified for each step, and a form of community evaluation is planned

Personal Awareness	
PS 6.5	Displays personal responsibility (time management, scheduling, problem solving, budgeting, decision making, etc.) [partial standard]
PS 7.3	Evaluates responsibility and consequences of choices and actions
PS 8.4	Strives for personal growth through commitment to lifelong learning
Goal Setting	
PS 6.5	Displays personal responsibility (time management, scheduling, problem solving, budgeting, decision making, etc.) [partial standard]
PS 7.3	Evaluates responsibility and consequences of choices and actions
PS 8.2	Makes informed decisions after exploring options and weighing consequences
PS 8.4	Strives for personal growth through commitment to lifelong learning
Steps for Success and Assessment: Problem Solving and Decision Making	
PS 6.2	Makes deadlines [partial standard]
PS 6.5	Displays personal responsibility (time management, scheduling, problem solving, budgeting, decisions making, etc.) [partial standard]

PS 7.1	Demonstrates ability to find community or continuing education resources (health clinics, city and tribal councils, employment services, trade school, college, etc.)
PS 7.3	Evaluates responsibility and consequences of choices and actions
PS 8.2	Makes informed decisions after exploring options and weighing consequences
PS 8.4	Strives for personal growth through commitment to lifelong learning
PS 8.5	Proposes strategies and support structures to assist in dealing with problems associated with family, school, and work

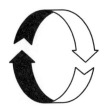

Systemic Renewal

Systemic renewal calls for a continuing process of evaluating goals and objectives related to school policies, practices, and organizational structures as they impact a diverse group of learners. Tools in this module include:

"How to Develop an Effective Dropout Prevention Program," developed by Teddy Holtz Frank, C.S.W., Hudson Valley Center for Coordinate School Health. Unpublished.

"How to Measure Your Organization's Progress," adapted from "Are We Making Progress?" National Institute of Standards and Technology, United States Department of Commerce, www.quality.nist.gov/progress.htm, copyright 2001.

How to Develop an Effective Dropout Prevention Program

 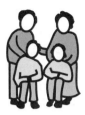   

In this section is an outline of an eight-step action planning process for creating an effective dropout prevention program. It details the specific steps and tools of the planning model designed for a school-based dropout prevention project (Destination: Graduation, sponsored by the New York State Education Department and implemented at Peekskill Middle School, New York, through the Hudson Valley Center for Coordinated School Health). It uses the framework of the principles of effectiveness as well as ecological intervention tools for creating and strengthening school–community partnerships. This model can be applied to the prevention of any risky youth behavior, such as substance use, early and unwanted pregnancy, human immunodeficiency virus/acquired immunodeficiency syndrome, violence, or—as it appears here—dropping out of school.

Eight Steps to Action Planning: A Process for Developing Effective Prevention Programs

An effective prevention programs must have as its foundation a thorough and complete analysis of the specific risk and protective factors that contribute to the formation of both the risk (i.e., "problem") behaviors as well as the healthy (i.e., "desired") behaviors.

Corresponding strategies to address the problem behaviors must be either research-based models or promising practices. These promising practices, although perhaps not yet rigorously evaluated, should be based on sound scientific theory. These strategies may be synonymous with identified protective factors, or they may be practical applications of these protective factors. For example, an identified risk factor when dealing with dropout prevention aimed at middle-school youth might be "lack of healthy role models of older youth." A protective factor would naturally be "healthy role models of older youth." A specific research-based strategy might be "a mentoring program that pairs high-school mentors with middle-school mentees." See the National Mentoring Partnership for additional resources on mentoring online at www.mentoring.org/index.adp.

Additionally, a strong working partnership between the school and the community must be established. This partnership increases available resources and acts as a significant protective factor by strengthening the safety net that keeps children from "falling through the cracks." The members responsible for implementing the action plan must be a cohesive, committed team of persons who represent the various sectors of that particular community. A key component for any effective planning process is the formation of this team.

Step 1: Creating a school–community team—community eco-map

Refer to the sections on "Who Should Be on the Action Team?" and "Eight Steps for Establishing an Action Team" and the eco-map on pages 130 and 133. Consult the following reference for further discussion on the use of this innovative tool for diagraming the human ecosystem within a community: Hartman A: Diagrammatic assessment of family relationships. *Social Casework* 59: 456–478, 1978.

Step 2: The vision process—creating a vision for the project

After each team member has had a chance to record his or her "vision," create a collective vision statement by incorporating all responses. This can take the form of a bulleted list or a narrative statement.

Step 3: Generating risk and protective factors

Present the Four Principles of Effectiveness. Consult the following reference for more information: United States Department of Education: *Non-regulatory Guidance for Implementing the Safe and Drug Free Schools and Community Act (SDFSCA) Principles of Effectiveness.* Washington, DC, United States Department of Education, Office of Elementary and Secondary Education, SDFSCA Program, May 1998.

Introduce the Needs Assessment process (Principle 1) as the analysis of risk and protective factors. This process is most effective when organized around data analysis using these five domains: individual and peer group, family, school, community, and sociopolitical environment (optional).

Using the worksheet on page 134, ask the group to generate the specific risk factors associated with students dropping out of high school for each of the domains. The last domain is optional because it can become more theoretical than practical. For each risk factor, identify indicators and corresponding data sources. See page 135 for an example of this process.

Using the worksheet on page 136, continue the process, matching risk factors with corresponding protective factors, effective research-based strategies, and promising programs. Indicate existing resources within the school and community, and identify any gaps in resources and services (see page 137 for an example of this process). Consult the following reference for promising practices and research-based strategies: Franklin S, Smink J: *Strategies to Help Solve Our School Dropout Problem.* West Larchmont, NY, Eye on Education, 2001.

Step 4: Narrowing the scope of the project—selecting risk factors

Ask the group to choose major risk factors from each of the domains. List one of them in each of the spaces in the first column of the worksheet on page 138. See page 139 for an example.

Step 5: Correlate research-based strategies and protective factors with selected risk factors

Using the same worksheet, match each of the selected risk factors with corresponding research-based strategies and protective factors from the previous handouts. See page 139 for an example.

Step 6: Generating goals and objectives for selected risk and protective factors

A goal is a broad statement of what is to be accomplished. The goals of the action plan should directly address what the earlier needs assessment process identified as being gaps in resources or services. Objectives detail the specific ways in which each goal will be achieved. Using the worksheet on page , list each goal and generate a list of corresponding objectives for each one, incorporating protective factors and research-based strategies into the objective. An example of this process is shown on page 141.

Step 7: Evaluation measures—performance indicators

An important part of this action-planning process is the periodic review and refinement of goals and objectives. Write up one or more performance indicators for each objective that detail how the accomplishment of this objective can be measured.

Step 8: Tasks and timelines

Break each objective into associated tasks and timelines for completion and associate it with the team member responsible for its accomplishment. This serves as a "map" to guide the team as they meet periodically. Each task can be checked for completion or revision along the way.

Who Should Be on the Action Team?

The action team, to be established by the school district, should be composed of 10 to 15 members who represent the following groups (members can be in more than one group):

- Middle school, high school, elementary school staff including principals, assistant principals, teachers, special educators, teachers union, guidance counselors, social workers, psychologists, and teacher aides
- Parents and guardians
- Youth and students
- District curriculum coordinators and administrators
- Board of Education members
- Community-based organizations
- Faith-based organizations
- Community and county agencies
- Business community
- Medical, health, and mental health agencies
- Social service agencies
- Higher education, universities, and community colleges

Eight Steps for Establishing an Action Team

Step 1: Identify who is currently a member of the local action team (LAT).

Identify what constituency (may be more than one) each member represents using the previous list of suggestions for persons who should compose the LAT.

Using the community eco-map (page 133), designate separate circles for each system, including elementary, middle, and high school. Write the name of the system in the circle. Write the role (i.e., social worker) of each member within his or her respective circle.

Draw a line between the LAT in the center of the eco-map and each of the circles to designate the nature of their connection. Use a solid line (_____) to denote a strong or solid connection to the LAT, a broken line (- - - - -) to denote a tenuous connection (e.g., a high school or elementary school principal not fully prepared for the job), and a railroad line (/\/\/\/\/\) to denote a problematic or adversarial connection (e.g., a school staff member negative toward any additional "work" or projects or who may actively try to block the efforts of the team).

Step 2: Brainstorm a list of *who* in the community is affected by the dropout problem.

Write down each system (e.g., family, business, law enforcement) that is not currently a member of the LAT within a separate circle on the eco-map.

Step 3: Discuss *how* each of these systems is affected by the dropout problem.

The results of this discussion can be listed next to each circle on the eco-map.

Step 4: **Link the *how* (i.e., way in which the systems are affected by the dropout problem) *with possible benefits* to each system of helping to solve the dropout problem within the community.** See page 141 for an example of the linking process.

Answer the critical question for each system. To put it another way, tune into station WIFM: What's In It For Me? In many instances, the benefits may simply be a matter of reversing costs.

Step 5: **Using the community eco-map, draw a broken line (- - - - -) from the LAT in the center, connecting any of these groups that should be represented but are not currently a part of the LAT.**

Step 6: **Identify a specific member within each group who can be contacted by a member of the LAT, and write their name in the circle.**

Step 7: **Designate who from the LAT might be the best person to contact each specific member of the groups listed on the community eco-map, and write their name above the dotted line.**

Discuss whom would be the person most likely to positively influence this system by factoring in previous relationship or connection, similarity of position or background, or ability to communicate favorably. Keep in mind the notion of WIFM, and look at it from the point of view of how involvement in the project can benefit the system.

Step 8: **Go back to the step one. Identify the weak or adversarial connections within the LAT.**

Apply the process outlined in steps three through seven to strengthen these connections within the team.

The Four Principles of Effectiveness

From "Non-regulatory Guidance for Implementing the Safe and Drug Free Schools and Community Act (SDFSCA) Principles of Effectiveness, United States Department of Education," Office of Elementary and Secondary Education, SDFSCA Program, May 1998.

◆ **Principle 1:** *Needs assessment*

A school district shall base its program on a thorough assessment of objective data about drug and violence problems in the schools and communities it serves.

◆ **Principle 2:** *Measurable goals and objectives*

A school district shall, with the assistance of a local or regional advisory council, establish a set of measurable goals and objectives and design its programs to meet these goals and objectives.

◆ **Principle 3:** *Research approaches to prevention*

School districts shall design and implement its programs for youth based on research and evaluation providing evidence that the programs used actually prevent or decrease drug use, violence, or disruptive behavior among youth.

◆ **Principle 4:** *Evaluation*

A school district shall evaluate its programs periodically to assess progress made toward achieving goals and objectives as well as use evaluation research to refine, improve, and strengthen its program and to refine goals and objectives as appropriate.

Community Eco-Map

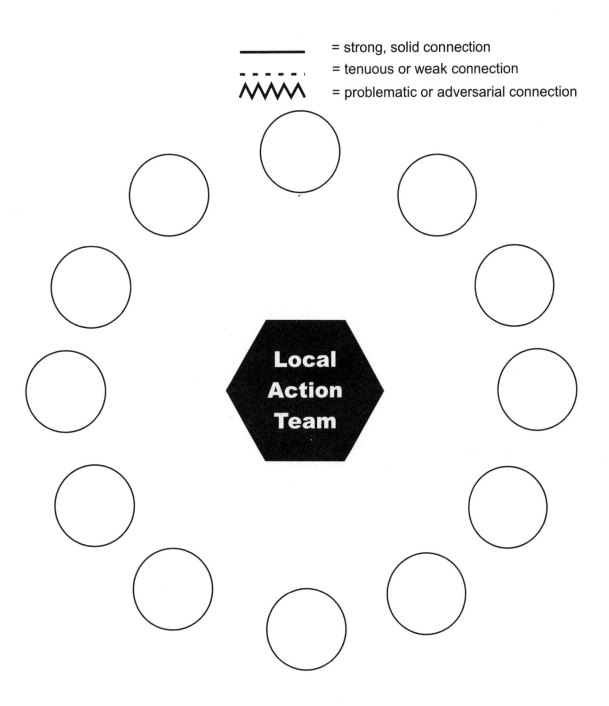

Handout for Generating Risk Factors

(Circle One)   Individual   Family   School   Community

Risk Factors	Indicators	Data Sources

Example of Risk Factors Generated by
Destination Graduation at Peekskill Middle School

(Circle one) (Individual)   Family   School   Community

Risk Factors	Indicators	Data Sources
Fighting and violence Substance abuse Promiscuity	Drug use, violence, provocative dress Talk and attitude favorable to drugs, sex, and violence	Violates school code of conduct, gets suspended and expelled Health care: sexually transmitted diseases, human immunodeficiency virus, injuries, drug overdose Juvenile justice and law enforcement: court and law enforcement involvement
Low expectations Disconnected and disaffected Low bonding to school Unrealistic goals Poor academic achievement	Poor test scores Drops out Does not complete assignments Poor grades	Test scores Report cards Attendance
Excessive family responsibilities Poverty and low socioeconomic status Lack of food, clean clothes, and school supplies	Misses school and homework assignments Tardy and/or leaves early No school supplies Does not attend school due to lack of clean clothes Has to care for younger siblings	Test scores Attendance Free and reduced-cost meals Department of Social Services

Handout to Correlate Risk Factors with Corresponding Protective Factors, Research-Based Strategies, and Programs

(Circle one)　(Individual)　Family　School　Community

Protective Factors	Resources

Example of Correlating Risk Factors with Corresponding Protective Factors, Research-Based Strategies, and Programs by Destination

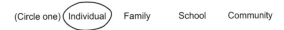

(Circle one) (Individual) Family School Community

Graduation at Peekskill Middle School

Protective Factors	*Community Resources*
(Correlated with risk factors) • Counseling and mental health strategies • Prevention curricula and skill building • Coordinated school health approaches • Mediation and conflict resolution • Law enforcement involvement and school resource officers • Clear and consistent communication of rules	• School counselors and community mental health counselors • Health teachers: prevention curricula • Hudson River Health Care Center: RAP Program (human immunodeficiency virus [HIV] and acquired immunodeficiency syndrome [AIDS] peer education), Girl Talk, Teen Clinic • Planned parenthood: health services, education abut sexually transmitted diseases and HIV • Youth Bureau programs • School resource officers • Positive behavioral intervention and support process (PBIS)
(Correlated with risk factors) • Connecting students' interest in photography, music, and art with academic areas and enrichment opportunities • Opportunities for youth involvement • Tutoring, homework help • Healthy adult and older youth role models • College preparation • Mentors, coaches, and advisors	• YES after-school program • Gear-Up (college preparation program at Westchester Community College) • Youth Bureau programs
(Correlated with risk factors) • Free and reduced-cost meals • Provide food, clothing, and school supplies • Provide referrals to community resources (to parents and guardians) for medical, housing, child care, food, employment, legal, and other services	• YES after-school program • Department of Social Services • Hudson River Health Care
(Integrates previous three areas) • Coordinate existing community programs with the school	• After-school and tutoring programs in Peekskill • Peekskill Agencies Together Meetings

Worksheet for Listing Risk Factors and Protective Factors

Risk Factor or Problem	*Protective Factors or Resources*

Example of Risk Factors and Protective Factors Generated by Destination: Graduation at Peekskill Middle School

Risk Factor or Problem

Protective Factors or Resources

Individual:

Students are disengaged from the school, resulting in poor attendance and grades

Individual:

Re-engage students through smaller group size (school within a school), mentoring programs, individualized attention and instruction, after-school programs, Gear Up, and family coordinators

Family:

Families lack access to resources such as food, clean clothing, adequate housing, child care, and employment, resulting in students having poor attendance and grades, possible behavior problems

Family:

Provide links to community resources for parents, and elicit parents' energy and involvement in child's education, family ties, EPIC Parent Program, community agencies, family coordinators

School:

Lack of differential instruction to accommodate all levels of students, resulting in wide achievement gap between students

School:

Staff development in differential instruction

Worksheet for Generating Goals and Objectives

Goal number:

Objectives:

Goal number:

Objectives:

Goals and Objectives Generated by Destination: Graduation at Peekskill Middle School

Goal no. 1:   Improve academic achievement for cohort of middle school students

Objectives:

1.   Develop criteria, and select 25 students to participate in pilot program to foster student achievement

2.   Develop and enhance leadership skills of a cohort of middle school students to build self-esteem

3.   Implement a variety of methods to celebrate student achievement to build self-esteem and ability to set and achieve goals

4.   Implement student orientation for cohort in collaboration with community-based organizations to engage students in program

5.   Implement mentoring program that partners high school and middle school students to ease the transition of middle schools students to high school

6.   Implement mentoring program that partners middle school and elementary school (incoming seventh-grade students) to develop leadership skills of middle school students and ease transition of sixth-grade students into middle school

7.   Implement adult and student mentoring program pairing cohort students with an adult mentor

8.   Facilitate participation in after-school program (YES) of cohort students to provide help with schoolwork and enrichment activities

9.   Supervise cohort participation in YES program and create strong links between school and YES program to furnish additional individualized help with school work and enrichment activities

10.   Begin planning process with Peekskill City School District to develop and implement training for school staff to integrate technology into classroom instruction.

References

Dynarski M, Gleason P: *How can we help? What we have learned from Evaluations of Federal Dropout-Prevention Programs*. Princeton, NJ: Mathematica Policy Research, 1998

Hartman A: Diagrammatic assessment of family relationships. *Social Casework* **59**: 456–478, 1978

Hawkins D, Catalano RF, Miller JY: 1992. Risk and protective factors for alcohol and other drug problems in adolescence and early adulthood: Implications for substance abuse prevention. *Psychology Bulletin* **112**(1): 64–105,

National Mentoring Partnership: Available at at: www.mentoring.org/index.adp (for additional resources on mentoring)

Schargel F, Smink J: *Strategies to Help Solve Our School Dropout Problem*. West Larchmont, NY: Eye On Education, 2001

United States Department of Education: *Non-regulatory Guidance for Implementing the Safe and Drug Free Schools and Community Act (SDFSCA) Principles of Effectiveness.* Washington, DC: United States Department of Education, Office of Elementary and Secondary Education, SDFSCA Program, May 1998

United States General Accounting Office: *School Dropouts: Education Could Play a Stronger Role in Identifying and Disseminating Promising Prevention Strategies.* Available at: www.gao.gov (click on "GAO reports" and enter report no. GAO-02-240)

How to Measure Your Organization's Progress

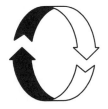  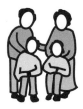  

The Malcolm Baldrige National Quality Award in Education is widely recognized as having devised a process to measure organizational excellence. The National Institute of Standards and Technology administers the Baldrige. They have developed the following questionnaire to help educational leaders measure organizational performance and learn what can be improved. As a result of completing this survey, the faculty might want to address the following questions:

- ♦ *Are the department's, school's, and district's vision, mission, values, and plans being deployed? How do you know?*
- ♦ *Are they understood by your leadership team? By the faculty? By the students? By the parents? How do you know?*
- ♦ *Are your communications effective? How do you know?*
- ♦ *Is your message being well received? How do you know?*

There are 40 statements below. For each statement, check the box that best matches how you feel (strongly disagree, disagree, neither agree or disagree, agree, strongly agree). How you will feel will help us decide where we most need to improve. We will not be looking at individual responses but will use the information from the entire group to make decisions. It should take approximately 10 to 15 minutes to complete this questionnaire.

Category 1: LEADERSHIP	Strongly Disagree	Disagree	Neither Agree nor Disagree	Agree	Strongly Agree
1a. I know my (choose one: department's, school's, district's) mission (what it is trying to accomplish).	☐	☐	☐	☐	☐
1b. My (choose one: supervisor's, principal's, superintendent's) use our organization's values to guide us.	☐	☐	☐	☐	☐
1c. My (choose one: supervisor's, principal's, superintendent's) creates a work environment that helps me do my job.	☐	☐	☐	☐	☐
1d. My (choose one: supervisor's, principal's, superintendent's) share information about the organization.	☐	☐	☐	☐	☐

Category 1: LEADERSHIP

	Strongly Disagree	Disagree	Neither Agree nor Disagree	Agree	Strongly Agree
1e. My (choose one: supervisor's, principal's, superintendent's) encourage learning that will help me advance my career.	☐	☐	☐	☐	☐
1f. My (choose one: department, school, district) lets me know what it thinks is most important.	☐	☐	☐	☐	☐
1g. My (choose one: department, school, district) asks what I think.	☐	☐	☐	☐	☐

Category 2: STRATEGIC PLANNING

2a. As it plans for the future, my (choose one: department, school, district) asks for my ideas.	☐	☐	☐	☐	☐
2b. I know the parts of my (choose one: department, school, district) plans that will affect me and my work.	☐	☐	☐	☐	☐
2c. I know how to tell if we are making progress on my (choose one: department's, school's, district's) goals and objectives.	☐	☐	☐	☐	☐

Category 3: STUDENT, STAKEHOLDER, AND MARKET FOCUS

(Note: your customers are the people who use the products of your work.)

3a. I know who my most important customers are.	☐	☐	☐	☐	☐
3b. I keep in touch with my customers.	☐	☐	☐	☐	☐
3c. My customers tell me what they need and want.	☐	☐	☐	☐	☐
3d. I ask if my customers are satisfied or dissatisfied with my work.	☐	☐	☐	☐	☐
3e. I am allowed to make decisions to solve problems for my customers.	☐	☐	☐	☐	☐

	Strongly Disagree	Disagree	Neither Agree nor Disagree	Agree	Strongly Agree

Category 4: INFORMATION AND ANALYSIS

	Strongly Disagree	Disagree	Neither Agree nor Disagree	Agree	Strongly Agree
4a. I know how to measure the quality of my work.	☐	☐	☐	☐	☐
4b. I know how to analyze (review) the quality of my work to see if changes are needed.	☐	☐	☐	☐	☐
4c. I use these analyses for making decisions about my work.	☐	☐	☐	☐	☐
4d. I know how the measure I use in my work fits into what the (choose one: department, school, district) is doing.	☐	☐	☐	☐	☐
4e. I get all the important information I need to do my work.	☐	☐	☐	☐	☐
4f. I get the information I need to know about how my (choose one: department, school, district) is doing.	☐	☐	☐	☐	☐

Category 5: FACULTY AND STAFF FOCUS

	Strongly Disagree	Disagree	Neither Agree nor Disagree	Agree	Strongly Agree
5a. I can make changes that will improve my work.	☐	☐	☐	☐	☐
5b. The people I work with cooperate and work as a team.	☐	☐	☐	☐	☐
5c. My (choose one: supervisor, principal superintendent) encourages me to develop my job skills so I can advance my career.	☐	☐	☐	☐	☐
5d. I am recognized for my work.	☐	☐	☐	☐	☐
5e. I have a safe workplace.	☐	☐	☐	☐	☐
5f. My (choose one: supervisor, principal superintendent's) and my ((choose one: department, school, district) care about me.	☐	☐	☐	☐	☐

	Strongly Disagree	Disagree	Neither Agree nor Disagree	Agree	Strongly Agree
Category 6: PROCESS MANAGEMENT					
6a. I can get everything I need to do my job.	☐	☐	☐	☐	☐
6b. I collect information (data) about the quality of my work.	☐	☐	☐	☐	☐
6c. We have good processes for doing our work.	☐	☐	☐	☐	☐
6d. I have control over my work processes.	☐	☐	☐	☐	☐
Category 7: ORGANIZATIONAL PERFORMANCE RESULTS					
7a. My customers are satisfied with my work.	☐	☐	☐	☐	☐
7b. My students meet all requirements.	☐	☐	☐	☐	☐
7c. I know how well my organization is doing.	☐	☐	☐	☐	☐
7d. My organization uses my time and talents well.	☐	☐	☐	☐	☐
7e. My organization removes things that get in the way of progress.	☐	☐	☐	☐	☐
7f. My organization obeys laws and regulations.	☐	☐	☐	☐	☐
7g. My organizations has high standards and ethics.	☐	☐	☐	☐	☐
7h. My organization helps me help my community.	☐	☐	☐	☐	☐
7i. I am satisfied with my job.	☐	☐	☐	☐	☐

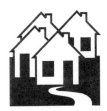

Community Collaboration

When all groups in a community provide collective support to the school, a strong infrastructure sustains a caring environment in which youth can thrive and achieve. Tools in this module include:

"How to Develop a Business Partnership Agreement," developed by Franklin P. Schargel. From "Transforming Education Through Total Quality Management: A Practioner's Guide," Eye On Education, 1994.

"How to Combat Truancy," adapted from "Manual to Combat Truancy," Prepared by the United States Department of Education in cooperation with the United States Department of Justice.

How to Develop a Business Partnership Agreement

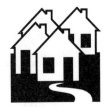 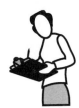 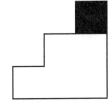

Many schools are involved with the business community, yet few have developed business partnership plans to help their business partners know what they need and want. What follows is one school's one business plan.

Dear business partner:

We would like you to consider helping us in the following ways:

- **Curriculum**

  Reviewing, revising, and developing curriculum so that graduating students will be trained to current standards.

- **Equipment**

  New, used, or broken but repairable and able to fit existing programs.

- **Jobs for Students**

  Co-op, after school, summer, and after graduation.

- **Paid Externships**

  For teachers to upgrade skills and create an awareness in students of what skills and qualities are needed in the business world.

- **Business Training Workshops**

  Workshops for teachers and students to learn techniques necessary for teaching employment skills (i.e., management, resume writing, computer programs).

- **Funds**

  Contributions to maintain and further develop existing programs and to provide college scholarships for graduating students.

- **Business People on Loan**

  Your people with expertise to speak to classes, to provide mock interviews, and to help with resume preparation.

Please return this form to:

Name: _____ School phone number: _____

How to Combat Truancy

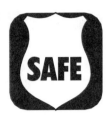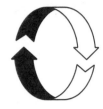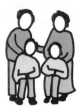

It stands to reason that a student who isn't in school learning will have a greater tendency to leave school before graduation. In addition, truancy is the most accurate predictor of juvenile delinquency. According to the Department of Juvenile Justice, in Miami more than 71% of 13- to 16-year-olds prosecuted for criminal violations had been truant. In Minneapolis, daytime crime decreased 68% after police began citing truant students. In Pittsburgh each day, approximately 3,500 students—or 12% of the pupil population—are absent, and approximately 70% of these absences are unexcused. In Philadelphia, approximately 2,500 students a day are absent without an excuse. In Chicago, 35,000 children are truant at least 1 day of the school year.

Truancy is a direct contributor to dropping out. Those who regularly do not attend school, do not regularly graduate. Each school needs to develop strategies, including a comprehensive strategy that focuses on incentives and sanctions for both truants and their parents, to deter truancy.

- ♦ **Involve parents in all truancy prevention activities.**

    Many truancy programs contain components that provide intensive monitoring, counseling, and other family-strengthening services to truants and their families. Schools may want to consider arranging convenient times and neutral setting for parent meetings, starting homework hotlines, training teachers to work with parents, hiring or appointing parent liaisons, and giving parents a voice in school decisions. In Milwaukee, Wisconsin, the Truancy Abatement and Burglary Suppression initiative calls parents at home automatically every night if their child did not attend school that day. If the parent is not supportive of regular school attendance, then the district attorney is contacted.

- ♦ **Ensure that students are aware they face firm sanctions for truancy.**

    State legislatures have found that linking truancy to student's grades or driver's licenses can help reduce the problem. Delaware, Connecticut and other states have daytime curfews during school hours that allow law enforcement officers to question youth to determine if their absence is legitimate.

- ♦ **Create meaningful incentives for parental responsibility.**

    It is critical that parents of truant children assume responsibility for truant behavior. It is up to each community to create meaningful incentives for such parents to ensure that their children get to school. In some states, parents of truant children are asked to participate in parenting education programs. Some other states, such as Maryland and Oklahoma, have determined that parents who fail to prevent truancy can be subject to formal sanction or lose eligibility for public assistance. There can also be *positive* incentives for responsible parents. Such incentives may include increased eligibility to participate in publicly funded programs. Local officials, educators, and parents working together can choose the incentives that make the most sense for their community. For example, Operation Safe Kids in Peoria, Arizona, contacts parents of students who have three unexcused absences. Parents are expected to relay back to school the official steps they have taken to ensure that their children regularly attend school. When children continue to be truant, cases are referred to the local district attorney. To avoid criminal penalty and a $150 parent fine, youth are required to participate in an intensive counseling program, and parents must attend a parenting skills training program.

◆ **Establish ongoing truancy prevention programs in school.**

Truancy can be caused by or related to such factors as drug use, violence at or near school or at home, association with truant friends, lack of family support for regular attendance, emotional or mental health problems, lack of a clear path to more education or work, or inability to keep pace with academic requirements. Schools must address the unique needs of each child and consider developing initiatives—including tutoring programs, added security measures, drug prevention initiatives, mentoring efforts through community and religious groups, campaigns for involving parents in their children's school attendance, and referrals to social serve agencies—to combat the root causes of truancy.

Schools need to find new ways to engage their students in learning, including such hands-on options as career academies, school-to-work opportunities, and service learning. They should enlist the support of local business and community leaders to determine the best way to prevent and decrease the incidence of truancy. For example, business and community leaders may lend temporary support by volunteering space to house temporary detention centers, by establishing community service projects that lead to after-school or weekend jobs, or by developing software to track truants. New Haven, Connecticut's Stay in School program targets middle school students who are sent to truancy court, at which a panel of high school students question them and try to identify solutions. After court, youth and attorney mentors are assigned to each student for support. The student and the court sign a written agreement and, after two months, students return to the court to review their contract and report their progress.

Students and parents in 10 elementary schools in Atlantic County, New Jersey's Project Helping Hand program with 5 to 15 days of unexcused absences meet with a truancy worker to provide short-term family counseling, up to 8 sessions. If a family fails to keep appointments, home visits are made to encourage cooperation. Once a truancy problem is corrected, the case is closed, and the truant student is placed on aftercare/monitoring status where contact made at 30-, 60-, and 90-day intervals to ensure that truancy does not persist. The Norfolk, Virginia, school district uses software to collect data on students who are tardy, who cut class and leave grounds without permission, who are truant but brought back to school by police, or who are absent without cause. School teams composed of teachers, parents, and school staff examine the data to analyze truancy trends. Marion Ohio's Community Service Early Intervention Program focuses on high school truants during their freshman year. Referred students are required to attend tutoring sessions and to give their time to community service projects and participate in a counseling program. In addition, students are required to give back to the Intervention Initiative by sharing what they have learned with new students in the program and by recommending others who might benefit. Parental participation is required throughout the program.

♦ **Involve local law enforcement in truancy reduction efforts.**

School officials should establish close links with local police, probation officers, and juvenile and family court officials. Police departments report favorably on community-run temporary detention centers where they can drop off truant youth rather than bring them to local police stations for time-consuming processing. Police sweeps of neighborhoods in which truant youth are often found can prove dramatically effective. The Stop, Cite, and Return Program of Rohnert Park, California, has patrol officers issue citations to suspected truants contacted during school hours, and students are returned to school to meet with their parents and a vice principal. Two citations are issued without penalty; the third citation results in referral to appropriate support services.

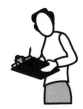

Career Education and Workforce Readiness

A quality guidance program is essential for all students. School-to-work programs recognize that youth need specific skills to prepare them for the larger demands of today's workplace. Tools in this module include:

"Identifying Workforce Skills and Competencies for the 21ˢᵗ Century: SCANS," from "What Work Requires of Schools: A SCANS Report for America 2000," United States Department of Labor, 200 Constitution Avenue, N.W., Washington, D.C. 20210, copyright, 2000.

"School-To-Work Continuum," developed by Franklin P. Schargel.

"Workforce Preparedness Quiz," developed by Roseann Cochran, Counselor, Rio Rancho High School, Rio Rancho, New Mexico.

Identifying Workforce Skills and Competencies for the 21st Century: The Secretary's Commission on Achieving Necessary Skills

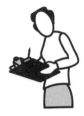  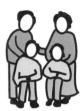  

During the course of its work, the United States Secretary of Labor appointed a group called the Secretary's Commission on Achieving Necessary Skills (SCANS), which produced several publications. Extensive meetings and discussions with a variety of organizations—including business, industry, public employers, and unions—resulted in the commission's first report, "What Work Requires of Schools." The report identifies 36 work place skills "that high-performance workplaces require and that high-performance schools should produce." These skills are divided into a three-part foundation and five competencies. The three-part foundation includes basic skills such as include literacy and computational skills, thinking skills described as necessary to put knowledge to work, and personal qualities described as making workers dedicated and trustworthy. The five competencies include the ability to manage resources, interpersonal skills needed to work amicably and productively with others, the ability to acquire and use information, skills needed to master complex systems, and skills needed to work with technology. It was the finding of the commission that these skills "lie at the heart of job performance and are essential preparation for all students, both those going directly to work and those planning further education." The commission believes that the most effective way of learning skills is "in-context" teaching, i.e., learning objectives within a real environment, and that the SCANS foundation and competencies should be taught and understood in an integrated fashion that reflects the workplace contexts in which they are applied.

Most children frequently fail to see the connection between what they learn in school and its relevance to the world of work. They question, "Why am I learning this?" In 1990, SCANS was appointed to determine the skills people need to succeed in the world of work. The commission was composed of 30 representatives of education, business, labor, and state government and was "charged with defining a common core of skills that constitute job readiness in the current economic environment.

The commission was asked to do the following:

- ◆ Define the skills needed for employment
- ◆ Propose acceptable levels of proficiency

- Suggest effective ways to assess proficiency
- Develop a dissemination strategy for the nation's schools, businesses, and homes.

Because the majority of students go into the world of work, it is important for them (including those at risk,) their parents, and their teachers to know what skills will be necessary for them to possess if they are to obtain meaningful employment.

The world continues to change as do the skills necessary for the workforce. Fewer than 50 years ago, "back power" jobs fuelled the economy. Today the economy is fueled by "brain power." At the beginning of World War II, students who did not complete high school were absorbed into the economy similar to those who did. Women could marry or become secretaries, teachers, or nurses. Men could work in factories, family farms, or the military. The factories of the industrial revolution are gone, replaced by high-technology industries that require thinking, problem-solving, team-organized members.

In 1991, the United States Department of Labor published the results of a study called SCANS (the Secretary's Commission on Achieving Necessary Skills.) The SCANS report delineated what the business community expected students to know and do to be successful in the workplace. Today it is more than critical to be aware of what the workplace requires from those entering it.

The SCANS report is broken down into a three-part foundation of skills and personal qualities with five areas of competencies.

Part One: Basic Skills

Reads, writes, performs arithmetic and mathematical operations, listens, and speaks.

- *Reading:* Locates, understands, and interprets written information in prose and in documents such as manuals, graphs, and schedules.
- *Writing:* Communicates thoughts, ideas, information, and messages in writing, and creates documents such as letters, directions, manuals, reports, graphs, and flow charts.
- *Arithmetic and mathematics:* Performs basic computations and approaches practical problems by choosing appropriately from a variety of mathematic techniques.
- *Listening:* Receives, attends to, interprets, and responds to verbal messages and other cues.
- *Speaking:* Organizes ideas and communicates orally.

Part Two: Thinking Skills

Thinks creatively, makes decisions, solves problems, visualizes, knows how to learn, and reasons.

- *Creative thinking:* Generates new ideas.
- *Decision making:* Sets specific goals and constraints, generates alternatives, considers risks, and evaluates and chooses best alternative.
- *Problem solving:* Recognizes problems and devises and implements plan of action.

- *Visualizes:* Organizes and processes symbols, pictures, objects, and other information.
- *Learns effectively:* Uses efficient learning techniques to acquire and apply new knowledge and skills.
- *Reasoning:* Discovers a rule or principle underlying the relationship between two or more objects and applies it when solving a problem.

Part Three: Personal Qualities

Displays responsibility, self-esteem, sociability, self-management, integrity, and honesty.

- *Responsibility:* Exerts a high level of effort and perseveres toward goal attainment.
- *Self-esteem:* Believes in own self-worth and maintains a positive view of self.
- *Sociability:* Demonstrates understanding, friendliness, adaptability, empathy, and politeness in group settings.
- *Self-management:* Assesses self accurately, sets personal goals, monitors progress, and exhibits self-control.
- *Integrity and honesty:* Chooses ethical courses of action.

Five Competencies

Competency One:

Resources (identifies, organizes, plans, and allocates resources)

- *Time:* Selects goal-relevant activities, ranks them, allocates time, and prepares and follows schedules.
- *Money:* Uses or prepares budgets, makes forecasts, keeps records, and makes adjustments to meet objectives.
- *Materials and facilities:* Acquires, stores, allocates, and uses materials or space efficiently.
- *Human resources:* Assesses skills and distributes work accordingly, evaluates performance, and provides feedback.

Competency Two:

Interpersonal (works well with others)

- *Participates as team member:* Contributes to group effort.
- *Teaches others new skills.*
- *Serves clients and customers:* Works to satisfy customer's expectations.
- *Exercises leadership:* Communicates ideas to justify position, to persuade and convince others, and to responsibly challenges existing procedures and policies.
- *Negotiates:* Works toward agreements involving exchange of resources and resolves divergent interests.

- *Works well in diverse environment:* Works well with people from diverse backgrounds.

Competency Three:

Information (acquires and uses information)
- *Acquires and evaluates information*
- *Organizes and maintains information*
- *Interprets and communicates information*
- *Uses computers to process information*

Competency Four:

Systems (understands complex interrelationships)
- *Understands systems:* Knows how social, organizational, and technological systems work and works effectively with them.
- *Monitors and corrects performance:* Distinguishes trends, predicts impacts on system operations, diagnoses systems' performance, and corrects malfunctions.
- *Improves or designs systems:* Suggests modifications to existing systems and develops new or alternative systems to improve performance.

Competency Five:

Technology (works with a variety of technologies)
- *Selects technology:* Chooses procedures, tools, or equipment, including computers and related technologies.
- *Applies technology to tasks:* Understands overall intent and proper procedures for setup and operation of equipment.
- *Maintains and troubleshoots equipment:* Prevents, identifies, or solves problems with equipment, including computers and other technologies.

School-to-Work Continuum

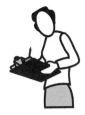 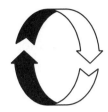  

At-risk children face the knowledge disadvantage because they have traditionally been concentrated in the most expendable job categories: low-skilled clerical and manufacturing jobs, which are destined for the greatest reductions in a technological economy. To prepare students for the world of work (page 160), what are the skills that schools need to teach them?

Elementary School (awareness)

Students in elementary school need to:

- ◆ Identify what work is
- ◆ Establish basic knowledge about what different occupations require
- ◆ Establish basic knowledge about different occupations
- ◆ Understand the concept of school as work
- ◆ Know about their own uniqueness
- ◆ Be acquainted with the relationship between money and work
- ◆ Understand the relationship between schoolwork and the world of work
- ◆ Recognize that their personal potential is limitless
- ◆ Understand that work values established in school are (e.g., preparedness, punctuality, and attendance) the foundation for success in the workplace

Middle School (exploration)

Students in middle school need to:

- ◆ Integrate career education into existing classroom curriculum
- ◆ Use guidance classes to promote career development.
- ◆ Use computerized career education delivery systems in the school library or public library.
- ◆ Focus on the importance of strong academic and vocational skill development
- ◆ Visit local, regional, and community college vocational programs

High School (preparation)

Students in high school need to:

- ◆ Develop occupationally specific skills
- ◆ Apply academic theory in real situations
- ◆ Master workplace basics

- Be trained and provided with appropriate information about jobs and career opportunities
- Develop a career plan
- Practice job shadowing and engage in real work experiences
- Connect work-based learning with school-based learning
- Engage in resume writing, interviewing skills training, and team-problem solving activities
- Engage in job shadowing and visits to industry, college, and vocational training institutions
- To assess interests and aptitudes

School-to-Work Continuum

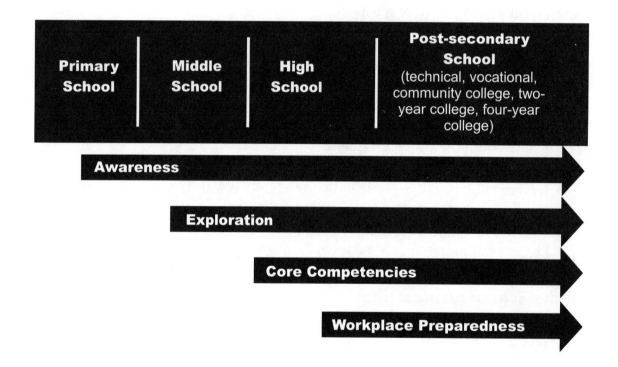

Workforce Preparedness Quiz

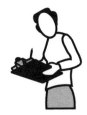 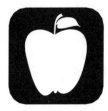 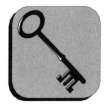 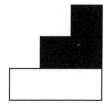

Many students do not connect what they learn in school with the world of work. This quiz will help them focus their energies.

Read the questions and options in each section, and think about the ones that sound like you. Ask your school counselor where you can get information about the fields that interest you.

Arts and Communication

Are you:

- a creative thinker?
- imaginative and innovative?
- original?
- a good communicator?

Do you:

- like to write?
- enjoy communicating ideas?
- use computers?
- enjoy performing?

With a high school diploma and some on-the job training, will you be a:

- floral arranger?
- display worker?
- model?
- cosmetics consultant?

Or with an associate's degree, technical or military training, will you be a(n):

- reporter?
- photographer?
- radio announcer?
- actor, singer, or dancer?
- graphic artist?

Or with a college degree, will you be a(n):

- designer?

- translator?
- advertising executive?
- editor or correspondent?
- Web master?

Business and Management

Are you:
- detail oriented?
- proficient with computers?
- organized?
- able to take on several tasks at one time?

Do you:
- like to organize people and projects?
- like to work with numbers and information?
- enjoy working in a business environment?
- get along well with people?

With a high school diploma and some on-the job training, will you be a:
- receptionist?
- postal clerk?
- bank teller?
- salesperson?

Or with an associate's degree, technical or military training, will you be a(n):
- court reporter?
- legal or medical secretary?
- administrative assistant?
- retail store manager?
- bookkeeper?

Or with a college degree, will you be a(n):
- computer programmer?
- executive or administrator?
- accountant or certified public accountant?
- loan officer?
- hotel manager?

Health and Medical Services

Are you:
- interested in science and research?
- compassionate?
- patient?

- observant?

Do you:

- like to care for the injured or sick?
- like to help people stay well?
- want to learn about new diseases?
- like to study how the body works?

With a high school diploma and some on-the job training, will you be a(n):

- home health aide?
- orderly or transporter?
- dental assistant?
- pharmacy clerk?
- dialysis technician?

Or with an associate's degree, technical or military training, will you be a(n):

- nurse?
- radiological technician?
- dental hygienist?
- emergency medical technician?
- respiratory therapist?

Or with a college degree, will you be a:

- physician or surgeon?
- physical therapist?
- pharmacist?
- psychiatrist?
- dentist?

Human and Public Services

Are you:

- friendly and outgoing?
- understanding?
- a good listener?
- patient?

Do you:

- like to help people solve their problems?
- want to make things better for other people?
- like talking with people?
- stay positive when times are tough?

With a high school diploma and some on-the job training, will you be a:

- preschool worker?
- recreation leader?

- teacher aide?
- food service worker?
- customs inspector?

Or with an associate's degree, technical or military training, will you be a:

- cosmetologist?
- fire fighter?
- police officer?
- corrections officer?
- chef?

Or with a college degree, will you be a:

- teacher?
- counselor?
- lawyer or judge?
- psychologist?
- social worker?

Engineering and Technology

Are you:

- mechanically inclined?
- interested in technology?
- inventive?
- practical and logical?

Do you:

- like to work with your hands?
- want to know how things work?
- like to design, put together, or build things?
- like to work with computers?

With a high school diploma and some on-the job training, will you be a:

- construction worker?
- carpenter?
- brick mason?
- highway maintenance worker?
- carpet installer?

Or…with an associate's degree, technical or military training, will you be a(n):

- mechanic?
- electrician?
- electronics technician?
- machinist?
- surveyor?

Or with a college degree, will you be a(n):

- aerospace engineer?
- city planner?
- computer engineer?
- architect?
- robotics engineer?

Natural Resources

Are you:

- a nature lover?
- curious about the physical world?
- concerned about the environment?
- interested in science?

Do you:

- enjoy being outside?
- like to travel?
- like to solve problems?
- like to raise or work with plants or animals?

With a high school diploma and some on-the job training, will you be a(n):

- groundskeeper or golf course caretaker?
- landscape worker?
- ranch hand?
- animal caretaker?

Or with an associate's degree, technical or military training, will you be a:

- veterinary lab assistant?
- chemical lab technician?
- metallurgical technician?
- pet store worker?

Or with a college degree, will you be a(n):

- meteorologist?
- astronomer?
- veterinarian?
- forester?
- conservationist?

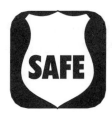

Safe Schools

A comprehensive violence prevention plan, including conflict resolution, must deal with potential violence as well as crisis management. Violence prevention means providing daily experiences at all grade levels that enhance positive social attitudes and effective interpersonal skills in all students. Tools in this module include:

"Key Findings Of The Safe School Initiative," adapted from "Threat Assessment in Schools: A Guide to Managing Threatening Situations and to Creating Safe School Climates," Washington, D.C., United States Secret Service and United States Department of Education, May 2002.

"How To Develop an In-School Suspension Plan Providing Structure for Disruptive Students," Jim F. Lawson, Mowat Middle School, Bay District Schools, Panama City, Florida; Copyright 2002, Jim Lawson, all rights reserved, used with permission.

"In-School Suspension Letter to Parents," developed by Franklin P. Schargel.

"How to Establish an Action Plan for School Leaders: Creating a Safe and Connected School Climate and Implementing a Threat Assessment Program," adapted from "Threat Assessment in Schools: A Guide to Managing Threatening Situations and to Creating Safe School Climates," Washington, D.C., United States Secret Service and United States Department of Education, May 2002.

"How To Evaluate a Truancy Reduction Project," adapted from "Evaluating a Truancy Reduction Demonstration Project," Washington, D.C., Office of Juvenile Justice and Delinquency Prevention, www.ojjdp.ncjrs.org.

"What Are the Predictors of Truancy?" adapted from the Kane County Truancy Prevention and Dropout Intervention Program Guidelines

"How to Identify a Teenager Who May Be Contemplating Suicide," adapted from the National Mental Health Awareness Campaign.

"**How to Prevent School Bullying,**" adapted from "Preventing Bullying: A Manual for Schools and Communities," Washington, D.C., United States Department of Education.

"**Establishing a School Safety Committee,**" developed by Franklin P. Schargel

"**Developing a School Safety Kit,**" developed by Franklin P. Schargel

Key Findings of the Safe School Initiative

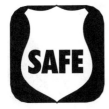 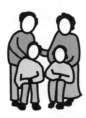  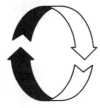 

There is nothing as frightening to school officials as the threat of school violence. Schools need to be sanctuaries of safety, although most schools were not designed that way. In reality, today's schools are still the safest places for children. According to a recent survey, 8 of 10 people interviewed believe that schools in their community are safe or very safe. In spite of that data, incidents like Columbine, Jonesboro, and West Paduca flash through the thoughts of parents, teachers, principals, and superintendents. It is easier to prevent school violence if we are aware of its warning signs. In the light of the spate of recent school violence, a large number of reports dealing with its prevention have been published. Following are some findings from those reports.

For students to achieve at the highest level possible, schools must be safe and secure so children can learn in an atmosphere free of fear and violence. Incidents of targeted school violence occurred in 37 communities across the United States between 1974 and 2000. Beginning in June 1999, the United States Department of Education and the United States Secret Service began working together to better understand and help to prevent school shootings in America. As a result, a series of publications has been issued through the Safe School Initiative, which issued "The Final Report and Findings of the Safe School Initiative: Implications for the Prevention of School Attacks in the United States and Threat Assessment in Schools: A Guide to Managing Threatening Situations and to Creating Safe School Climates." The focus of threat assessment is on prevention, not on resolution.

The 10 key findings of the Safe School Initiative are as follows:

- ◆ Incidents of targeted violence at school rarely are sudden, impulsive acts.
- ◆ Before most incidents occur, other people often know about the attacker's idea and/or plan to attack.
- ◆ Most attackers do not threaten their targets directly before making the attack.
- ◆ There is no accurate or useful "profile" of students who engage in targeted school violence.
- ◆ Most attackers were known to have difficulty coping with significant losses or personal failures. Many had considered or attempted suicide before attacking.
- ◆ Many attackers felt bullied, persecuted, or injured by others before attacking.
- ◆ Most attackers had access to and had used weapons before the attack.
- ◆ In many cases, other students were involved in some capacity.
- ◆ Despite prompt law enforcement responses, most shooting incidents are stopped by means other than law enforcement intervention.

How to Develop an In-School Suspension Plan Providing Structure for Disruptive Students

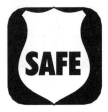 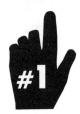 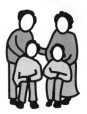 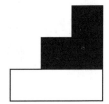

Students need structure, and at-risk students need more structure than most. Schools must supply that structure so all students can succeed and thrive in school and the larger world. Students who disrupt classes not only deprive themselves but others as well. Suspending students makes little sense; it frequently gives them the attention they crave and "permission" to take time off from learning. On the other hand, allowing them to remain in class, possibly to disrupt again, fails to show them the negative consequences of their actions. In-school suspension (ISS) provides the best of both worlds by supplying students with the structure that may be lacking outside the school building. At-risk students frequently need more structure with clearly delineated limits.

The Assessment Tool

Creating an instrument for measuring student performance is the core of any approach to achieving effective classroom management. One such measurement tool is a rubric designed to assess the behavior of students assigned to an ISS class. Each ISS student is assigned a score, using a "0-to-5" scale, to measure his or her level of performance on each of five separate criteria. These standards for assessment are important for any classroom teacher or program administrator: attendance, tardiness, ability to follow rules and policies, behavior, and on-task or off-task behavior.

When a student assigned to ISS scores "0" points, he or she has successfully completed the in-school requirements in a "superior" manner. A student who scores "1 to 4" points has successfully completed the in-school requirements but "needs to improve" in one or more of the criterion areas. Finally, the student who scores "5 or more" points, "did not successfully complete" the ISS requirements and is reassigned to an out-of-school suspension. Students who are assigned to ISS are allowed a maximum of "5" points regardless of the length of suspension. It should be noted that every student has the opportunity to start and finish each in-school suspension assignment with "0" points.

As an assessment tool the application of this rubric allows the following:

♦ Consistent enforcement for inappropriate behavior or rules violations

♦ A way for students to monitor their behavior and performance

- A way for students to calculate their probability for success
- Fairness and flexibility from the program's administrator
- Administrative support for the process and the program administrator

The design of this rubric may be edited or revised to meet the needs of any school, teacher, classroom, or program.

Rubric for Assessing In-School Suspension Performance

Student performance level is assessed on a scale of "0" to "5": "0" = superior; "1" = average; "2" = needs improvement; "3" = unsatisfactory behavior; "4" = warning of dismissal; "5" = dismissal.

Criteria For Assessment*	0 Points +	1 Point	2 Points	3 Points	4 Points	5 Points
Off-task behavior	On-task	Off-task	Off-task	Off-task	Off-task	Off-task
Disruptive behavior	No disruptive behavior	Disruptive behavior	Disruptive behavior	Disruptive behavior	Disruptive behavior	Disruptive behavior
Rules and policies	Followed all rules	Violated rules	Violated rules	Violated rules	Violated rules	Violated rules
Unexcused tardiness	No tardy	First tardy	Second tardy	Third tardy	Fourth tardy	Fifth (or more) tardy
Books and/or materials	Books and/or materials	No books and/or materials	No books and/or materials	No books and/or materials	No books and/or materials	No books and/or materials
Dress code	Dress code violation	Dress code violation	Dress code violation	Dress code violation	Dress code violation	Dress code violation
*What I'm looking for; + the level at which my students need to perform.						

In-School Suspension
Letter to Parents

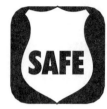 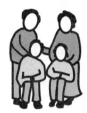 

Schools find that having "time-out rooms" are more effective than out-of-school suspensions. These rooms allow students to "cool down" and contemplating the ramifications of their behavior. Students can be sent to the room for several days, a few hours, or even for the one class period during which they were disruptive. Parents need to be notified of the infraction. Below is a sample letter to be sent to parents. Feel free to modify it to suit your school's needs.

Date

Dear Parent or Guardian:

This letter is to inform you that your child

was placed in the in-school suspension room for:

One class   Hour(s)

Day(s)

The reason for this in-school suspension was:

☐ Disruptive conduct   ☐ Tardiness

☐ Improper language   ☐ Bullying

☐ Disrespect to teachers   ☐ Harassment

Other:

If your child's behavior does not improve, we will be forced to suspend him/her from school in accordance with school and district regulations. If you would like to speak to me or have any questions, I can be reached at

Sincerely,

Dean

Principal

How to Establish an Action Plan for School Leaders: Creating a Safe and Connected School Climate and Implementing a Threat Assessment Program

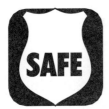 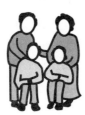   

Some schools' culture and climate can contribute to the prevention of violence. How does a school, its teachers and administrators, and its students work toward implementing a culture of safety?

Major Components and Tasks for Creating a Safe and Connected School Climate

♦ Assess the school's emotional climate.

It is incumbent on those in positions of authority and responsibility to assess the emotional climate of their school. This perspective can be gained by systematically surveying students, faculty, parents, administrators, school board members, and representatives of community groups about the emotional climate of schools. Anonymous surveys, face-to-face interviews, focus groups, and school climate surveys allow school officials to gather valuable insights about the school's emotional climate.

♦ Emphasize the importance of listening in schools.

A school with a culture of "two-way listening" encourages and empowers students to break the ingrained code of silence. Listening also must be expanded beyond academic concerns. Communication between teachers and students should also include listening to feelings, especially those of hurt and pain. It is also important to "listen" to behaviors. Many students have a difficult time finding the words to articulate disenfranchisement, hurt, or fear.

♦ Take a strong, but caring, stance against the code of silence.

Silence leaves hurt unexposed and unacknowledged. Silence may encourage a young person to move along a path to violence.

♦ Work to change the perception that talking to an adult about a student contemplating violence is considered "snitching."

- Find ways to stop bullying.

  Bullying is a continuum of abuse ranging from verbal taunts to physical threats to dangerous acts. Bullying is not playful behavior. In bullying, one student assumes power by word or deed over another in a mean-spirited and/or harmful manner. Schools must establish climates of safety and respect, which establish foundations for prosocial behavior. These climates teach conflict resolution, peer mediation, active listening, and other nonviolent ways to solve problems. In a safe school climate, adults do not bully students and do not bully each other, and they do not ignore bullying behavior when they know that it is going on in the school.

- Empower students by involving them in planning, creating, and sustaining a school culture of safety and respect.

  Creating a climate of safety should be a collaborative effort.

- Ensure that every student feels that he or she has a trusting relationship with at least one adult at school.

  These trusting relationships evolve and do not magically appear simply because an adult, such as a homeroom teacher or a guidance counselor, and a student have been ordered or assigned to interact with one another.

- Create mechanisms for developing and sustaining safe school climates.

  A mechanism for developing and sustaining safe school climates should serve as a vehicle for planning and monitoring the climate and culture of the school. Questions to be considered in implementing this mechanism might include the following: What should be done to develop and support climates of safety? To what extent are teachers, administrators, and other school staff encouraged to focus on students' social and emotional learning needs? How close is the school to achieving the goal of ensuring that every student feels that there is an adult to whom he or she can turn for talk, support, and advice if things get tough?

- Be aware of physical environments and their effects on creating comfort zones.

  Building structure, facility safety plans, lighting, space, and architecture—among other physical attributes of educational institutions—can contribute to whether a school environment feels, or is in fact, safe or unsafe. In large schools, administrators may wish to explore changes in the physical characteristics of the school that would permit the assignment of teachers and students to smaller, mutually intersecting and supportive groupings within the larger physical structure.

- Emphasize an integrated systems model.

  People support most what they believe they have had genuine input in creating. This requires the difficult but necessary task of bringing all of the stakeholders to bear on changes made for safety. Stakeholders include students, teachers, administers, school board members, parents, law enforcement personnel, after-school and community-based groups, and others.

♦ All climates of safety ultimately are "local."

Many local factors contribute to the creation of a culture and climate of safety. These factors include the following:

- Leadership, i.e., "open door" role of the school principal
- "Empowered buy-in" of student groups
- Connections to the local community and its leaders
- Respectful integration into the safe school climates process of "safekeepers," such as parents and law enforcement personnel close to the school

How to Evaluate a Truancy Reduction Project

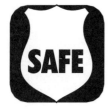

The Office of Juvenile Justice and Delinquency Prevention sets evaluation guidelines to evaluate the success of its truancy reduction programs. By providing answers to the questions below, designers of school or district programs will understand the most important components for the success of grants and projects.

- ◆ What needs are being addressed by the project?
- ◆ How do all aspects of each project form a coherent strategy?
- ◆ How is truancy identified?
- ◆ What systems are in place to ensure an accurate count of truants as defined in the background section?
- ◆ What collaborative ties have been developed, and what purpose do they serve?
- ◆ How does each project relate to larger community goals and visions?
- ◆ Do youth have opportunities to exercise responsibility for parts of the project? Are there opportunities for young people to make suggestions to improve or modify program activities? How does the program respond?
- ◆ How are youth provided with information and access to additional services and support such as mental, physical, recreational, and cultural services?
- ◆ How does the project involve families and peers?
- ◆ How is the project sensitive to the cultural diversity of its clients? How do project activities promote cultural awareness?
- ◆ What factors influence effective implementation of a truancy reduction program? (Special attention should be paid to the problems encountered in implementing the truancy reduction project in collaboration with other programs already under way within communities.)
- ◆ What changes, such as changes in attitudes among stakeholder agencies, have resulted from implementation of the project?
- ◆ What factors contribute to the institutionalization of a collaborative truancy reduction program within the communities?
- ◆ What planning and implementation strategies (e.g., coordination, consultation, use of OJP-provided technical assistance) are used at local levels, and what is the effect of their use?

What Are the Predictors of Truancy?

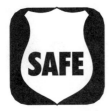 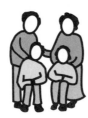  

Certain factors correlate with truancy, which correlates with dropping out. The Kane County School System of Geneva, Illinois, has identified 27 such factors.

Predictors of Future Truancy

- Attendance patterns: frequent absences, suspicious excuses from school, frequent tardiness
- Poor classroom performance
- Peer relationships: loner, fights, not chosen for games, shy
- Limited participation in extracurricular activities and physical education
- Physical appearance: dress, personal hygiene, size, health
- Eating disorders: anorexia, bulimia, obesity
- Sibling performance in school was negative, or sibling dropout out is or was truant
- Family environment reveals problems (e.g., overprotected)
- Two or more years behind in reading and/or mathematics
- Failure of one or more school years in elementary school
- Friends not school oriented or dropouts/truants
- Friends much older and/or substance abusers
- Behavior problems requiring disciplinary measures
- Recent divorce in the home or single-parent home
- Alcohol and/or drug abuse and/or child of alcoholic family system
- Emotional problems/psychosomatic illness, asthma, colitis, ulcers, eczema, enuresis, encorpresis
- Absent from home without parental consent
- Recent death in the home or terminally ill parent
- Lack of parental supervision before and/or after school
- Abused and/or neglected (spouse and/or child)
- Disconnected or no phone during the last school year
- Behavior disorder or learning disorder placement
- Moved four or more times during elementary school period
- Twenty or more absences in kindergarten or first grade
- Separation issue of parent and/or child
- Frequent change of schools
- Feelings of not belonging and social isolation

How to Identify a Teenager
Who May Be Contemplating Suicide

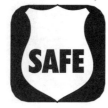  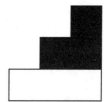

Five thousand teenagers and young adults commit suicide each year. Many teenagers say they know a teenager who has attempted or committed suicide. Children who are at-risk may feel under increased pressure to contemplate the act. What do schools need to watch for in identifying teens showing early warning signs of suicide?

Signs That a Teenager May Be Contemplating Suicide

♦ Depression
♦ Change in eating habits and sleep patterns
♦ Falling grades
♦ Anxiety or panic
♦ Lack of interest in activities normally enjoyed
♦ Decreased interaction with friends
♦ Giving away personal items
♦ Withdrawal from family
♦ Increase in alcohol or drug consumption
♦ Family history of suicide
♦ Anger or self-destructive behavior
♦ Talking about death or dying
♦ Previous suicide attempt

How to Prevent School Bullying

 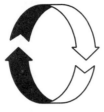 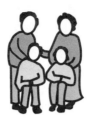  

Because of the recent incidents of school violence, bullying has become a matter of concern for a number of school stakeholders. In a study conducted in small Midwestern towns, 88% of students reported having observed bullying, and 76.8% indicated they had been a victim of bullying. Of the nearly 77% who had been victimized, 14% indicated that they experience severe reactions to the abuse. A study of 6,500 fourth- to sixth-graders in the rural South indicated that 1 in 4 students had been bullied with some regularity and that 1 in 10 had been bullied at least once a week. Bullying can lead to greater and prolonged violence. Not only does it harm its intended victims, it also negatively affects school climate and opportunities for all students to learn and achieve in school.

What Is Bullying?

Bullying among children is commonly defined as intentional, repeated hurtful acts, words or other behavior—such as name calling, threatening, and/or shunning—committed by one or more children against another. Bullying may be physical, verbal, emotional, or sexual in nature. For example:

- Physical bullying includes punching, poking, strangling, hair pulling, beating, biting, and excessive tickling.
- Verbal bullying includes hurtful name-calling, teasing, and gossip.
- Emotional bullying includes rejecting; terrorizing; extorting; defaming; humiliating; blackmailing; rating or ranking of personal characteristic such as race, disability, ethnicity, or perceived sexual orientation; manipulating friendships; isolating; ostracizing; and peer pressure.
- Sexual bullying includes many of the actions listed above as well as exhibitionism, voyeurism, sexual propositioning, sexual harassment, and abuse involving actual physical contact and sexual assault.

Who Gets Hurt?

Victims can suffer far more than actual physical harm.

- Grades may suffer because attention is drawn away from learning.
- Fear may lead to absenteeism, truancy, or dropping out.
- Victims may lose or fail to develop self-esteem, experience feelings of isolation, and become withdrawn and depressed.

- As students and later as adults, victims may be hesitant to take social, intellectual, emotional, or vocational risks.
- If the problem persists, victims occasionally feel compelled to take drastic measures, such as vengeance in the form of fighting back, weapon carrying, or even suicide.
- Victims are more likely than nonvictims to grow up being socially anxious and insecure, displaying more symptoms of depression than those who were not victimized as children.
- Bystanders and peers of victims can be distracted from learning as well.
- They may be afraid to associate with the victim for fear of lowering their own status or of retribution from the bully and becoming victims themselves.
- They may fear reporting bullying incidents because they do not want to be called a "snitch," a "tattler," or an "informer."
- They may experience feelings of guilt or helplessness for not standing up to the bully on behalf of their classmate.
- They may feel unsafe, unable to take action, or out of control.

Bullies attend school less frequently and are more likely to drop out of school than other students. Several studies suggest that bullying in early childhood may be an early sign of the developing of violent tendencies, delinquency, and criminality.

Developing a Comprehensive Approach

School-Level Interventions

- Develop a student questionnaire to determine the nature and extent of bullying problems in school.
- Formation of a bullying prevention coordinating committee (a small group of energetic teachers, administrators, counselors, and other school staff who plan and monitor school activities.)
- Hold teacher in-service days to review findings from the questionnaire, discuss bullying problems, and plan the school's violence prevention efforts.
- Sponsor schoolwide events to launch the program (e.g., via school television, public address announcements, or assemblies.)
- Develop schoolwide rules and sanctions against bullying.
- Develop a system to reinforce prosocial behavior (e.g., "Caught you Caring" initiatives).
- Involve parents school activities (e.g., highlighting the program at Parent-Teacher Association meetings, school open houses, and special violence prevention programs; encourage parents' participation in planning activities and school events).
- Schedule regular classroom meetings during which students and teachers engage in discussion, role playing and artistic activities related to preventing bullying and other forms of violence among students.

Individual Interventions

♦ School staff members intervene immediately in all bullying incidents.

♦ When appropriate, involve parents of bullies and victims of bullying are involved.

♦ Form "friendship groups," or other supports for students who are victims of bullying.

♦ When appropriate, involve school counselors and/or mental health professionals.

Community Interventions

♦ Disseminate information about the program known among a wide range of residents in the local community (e.g., convene meetings with community leaders to discuss the school's program and problems associated with bullying, encourage local media coverage of the school's efforts, engage students in efforts to discuss their school's program with informal community leaders).

♦ Involve community members in the school's antibullying activities (e.g., solicit assistance from local businesses to support aspects of the program, involve community members in school and districtwide "Bully-Free Day" events).

♦ Engage community members, students, and school personnel in antibullying efforts within the community (e.g., introduce core program elements into summer church school classes).

Before implementing any efforts to address bullying or other violence at school, school administrators should keep in mind the following:

♦ Ideally, efforts should begin early, as children transition into kindergarten, and continue throughout a child's formal education.

♦ Effective programs require strong leadership and ongoing commitment on the part of school personnel.

♦ Ongoing staff development and training are important to sustaining programs.

♦ Programs should be culturally sensitive to student diversity issues and developmentally appropriate.

♦ Parent and community involvement in the panning and execution of such programs is critical.

Administrative Interventions

♦ Assess the awareness and the scope of the bullying problems at school through student and staff surveys.

♦ Closely supervise children on playgrounds and in classrooms, hallways, rest rooms, cafeterias, and other areas where bullying occurs in school.

♦ Conduct schoolwide assemblies and teacher and staff in-service training to raise awareness regarding the problem of bullying and to communicate zero tolerance for such behavior.

- Post and publicize clear behavior standards, including rules against bullying, for all students. Consistently and fairly enforce such behaviors.

- Encourage parent participation by establishing on-campus parent centers that recruit, coordinate, and encourage parents to take part in the educational process and volunteer to assist in school activities and projects.

- Establish a confidential reporting system that allows children to report victimization and that records the details of bullying incidents.

- Ensure that your school has legally required policies and procedures for sexual discrimination. Make these procedures known to parents and students.

- Receive and listen receptively to parents who report bullying. Establish procedures whereby such reports are investigated and resolved expeditiously at the school level to avoid perpetuating bullying.

- Develop strategies to reward students for positive, inclusive behavior.

- Provide schoolwide and classroom activities designed to build self-esteem by spotlighting special talents, hobbies, interests, and abilities of all students and that foster mutual understanding of and appreciation for differences in others.

Teacher Interventions

- Provide students with opportunities to talk about bullying, and enlist their support in defining bullying as unacceptable behavior.

- Involve students in establishing classroom rules against bullying. Such rules may include a commitment from the teacher to not "look the other way" when incidents involving bullying occur.

- Provide classroom activities and discussions related to bullying and violence, including the harm that they cause and strategies to reduce their incidence.

- Develop a classroom action plan to ensure that students know what to do when they observe a bully–victim confrontation.

- Teach cooperation by assigning projects that require collaboration. Such cooperation teaches students how to compromise and how to assert without demanding. Take care to vary grouping of participants and to monitor the treatment of and by participants in each group.

- Take immediate action when bullying is observed. All teaches and school staff must let children know they care and will not allow anyone to be mistreated. By taking immediate action and dealing directly with the bully, adults support both the victim and the witnesses.

- Confront bullies in private. Challenging bullies in front of their peers may actually enhance their status and lead to further aggression.

- Notify parents of both victims and bullies when a confrontation occurs, and seek to resolve the problem expeditiously at school.

- Refer both victims and aggressors to counseling when appropriate.

- Provide protection for bullying victims when necessary. Such protection may include creating a buddy system whereby students have a particular friend or older buddy on whom they can depend and with whom they share class schedule information and plans for the school day.

- ♦ Listen receptively to parents who report bullying, and investigate reported circumstances so immediate and appropriate school action may be taken.
- ♦ Avoid attempts to mediate a bullying situation. The difference in power between victims and bullies may cause victims to feel further victimized by the process or to believe they are somehow at fault.

Student Interventions

Students may not know what to do when they observe a classmate being bullied or experience such victimization themselves. Classroom discussions and activities may help students develop a variety of appropriate actions that they can take when they witness or experience such victimization. For instance, depending on the situation and their own level of comfort, students can do the following:

- ♦ Seek immediate help from an adult and report bullying and victimization incidents to school personnel
- ♦ Speak up and/or offer support to the victim when they see him or her being bullied (e.g., picking up the victim's books and handing them to him or her)
- ♦ Privately support those being hurt those being hurt with words of kindness or condolence
- ♦ Express disapproval of bullying behavior by not joining in the laughter, teasing, or spreading of rumors or gossip
- ♦ Attempt to defuse problem situations either single handedly or in a group (e.g., by taking the bully aside and asking him or her to "cool it"

Parent Interventions

The best protection parents can offer their children who are involved in a bully–victim conflict is to foster their child's confidence and independence and to be willing to take action when needed. The following suggestions are offered to help parents identify appropriate responses to conflict experienced by their children at school:

- ♦ Be careful not to convey to a child who is being victimized that something is wrong with him or her or that he or she deserves such treatment. When a child is subjected to abuse from his or her peers, it is not fair to fault the child's social skills. Respect is a basic right: All children are entitled to courteous and respectful treatment. Convince your child that he or she is not at fault and that the bully's behavior is the source of the problem.
- ♦ It is appropriate to call the school if your child is involved in a conflict as either a victim or a bully. Work collaboratively with school personnel to address the problem. Keep records of incidents so that you can be specific in your discussion with school personnel about your child's experiences at school.
- ♦ You may wish to arrange a conference with a teacher, principal, or counselor. School personnel may be able to offer some practical advice to help you or your child. They may also be able to intervene directly with each of

the participants. School personnel may have observed the conflict first-hand and may be able to corroborate your child's version of the incident, making it harder for the bully or the bully's parents to deny its authenticity.

♦ Although it is often important to talk with the bully or his or her parents, be careful in your approach. Speaking directly to the bully may signal to the bully that your child is a weakling. Speaking with the parents of a bully may not accomplish anything because lack of parental involvement in a bullying child's life is typical. Parents of bullies may also fail to see anything wrong with bullying, equating it to "standing up for oneself."

♦ Offer support to your child, but do not encourage dependence on you. Rescuing your child from challenges, or assuming responsibility yourself when things are not going well, does not teach your child independence. The more choices a child has to make, the more he or she develops independence, and independence can contribute to self-confidence.

♦ Do not encourage your child to be aggressive or to strike back. Chances are that it is not his or her nature to do so. Rather, teach your child to be assertive. A bully often is looking for an indication that his or her threats and intimidation are working. Tears or passive acceptance only reinforces the bully's behavior. A child who does not respond as the bully desires is not likely to be chosen as a victim. For example, children can be taught to respond to aggression with humor and assertions rather than acquiescence.

♦ Be patient. Conflict between children more than likely will not be resolved overnight. Be prepared to spend time with your child, encouraging your child to develop new interests or strengthen existing talents and skills that will help develop and improve his or her self-esteem. Also help your child to develop new or bolster existing friendships. Friends often serve as buffers to bullying.

♦ If the problem persists or escalates, you may need to seek an attorney's help or contact local law enforcement officials. Bullying or acts of bullying should not be tolerated in the school or the community. Students should not have to tolerate bullying at school any more than adults would tolerate such situations at work.

Establishing a School Safety Committee

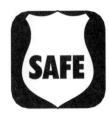  

Schools were not built with safety in mind. Many schools have "hidden" entrances and stairwells. All schools should develop a school safety committee to prepare to deal with school violence and, more importantly, to prevent its occurrence.

Mission:

♦ To promote and keep the school safe and secure

Members:

♦ One school administrator, three or fewer staff members concerned with school safety, one parent representative

Outside Resources Available:

♦ Police, fire department, emergency medical services, local hospital, community resources

Role of School Safety Committee

♦ Create a vision of a safe school
♦ Do a "security walk" through the school building looking for hidden entrances and stairwells and points of weakness where an intruder might enter without being stopped or identified
♦ Publicize efforts to staff, students, parents, and community

Developing a School Safety Kit

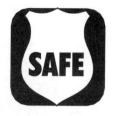  

Sometimes the school may have to be evacuated. Sometimes, the students and faculty must remain outside the building for an extended period of time. Each classroom should have a safety kit with adequate supplies to aid students, parents, and faculty in the event of an extended period spent outside the school building.

Suggested Contents of the School Safety Kit

Towels	Safety pins
Masking tape	Plastic bucket
Sealable plastic bags	Bandages
Cotton gloves	Plastic and rubber gloves
Name tags	Plastic cups
First aid kit	Permanent markers
Pencils	Wet wipes
Sunglasses	Hard candy
Umbrella	Sunscreen
Large plastic bags	Small plastic bags
Whistle	Tweezers
Duct tape	Waterless soap

Emergency contact cards with students' names, addresses, and phone numbers

Emergency phone numbers for police, fire department, local hospital, school superintendent

List of Contributors

The Afterschool Corporation (TASC), 925 Ninth Avenue, New York, HY 10019, info@tascorp.org, 212-547-6950

American YouthWorks Charter School, Lois Myers, Curriculum Specialist, Austin, TX 78701, 512-236-6150

Linda Borsum, Quality Learning Systems International, 4950 West Dickman Road, Suite B-3, Battle Creek, Michigan 49015; 800-379-2322, www.qlsi.com, used with permission

Jim Campbell, Performance Unlimited, www.Performance.Unlimited.com, 505-292-8832

Dr. John V. "Dick" Hamby, 216 West Academy Street, Kingstree, SC 29556

Chugash School District, Richard DeLorenzo, Superintendent; Debbie Treece, Quality Schools Coordinator, 9312 Vanguear Drive, No. 100, Anchorage, Alaska 99507 (704) 907-7400, www.chugashschools.com

Roseann Cochran, Counselor, Rio Rancho High School, Rio Rancho, New Mexico

R. Fein, B. Vossekuil, W. Pollack, R. Borum, W. Modzeleski, and M. Reddy: *Threat Assessment in Schools: A Guide to Managing Threatening Situations and to Creating Safe School Climates.* Washington, DC: United States Secret Service and United States Department of Education, published May 2002

Teddy Holtz Frank, C.S.W., New York State's Hudson Valley Center for Co-ordinated School Health, tfrank@mhric.org, 845-255-4874

Kane County Schools, Clem Mejia, Regional Superintendent; Pat Dal Santo, Director; Sandy Kakacek, Family Counselor; 210 South 6th Street, Geneva, IL 60134, 630-232-5955, Kane County Truancy Prevention/Dropout Intervention Program

Dr. Jim Kavanaugh and Kenneth J. Carson, material adapted from *Everyday Heroes: A Guidebook for Mentors* by Jim Kavanaugh, Ph.D., based on the Wise Men and Women Mentorship Program, Kenneth J. Carson, Sr., Founder and Director

Jim F. Lawson, Mowat Middle School, Bay District Schools, Panama City, Florida Located in Lynn Haven

Lonnie L. Leland, Program Coordinator and Becky LaVey, M.S.W., Program Social Worker, Project Transition, Bryan Station Traditional High School, 1866 Edgeworth Drive, Lexington, Kentucky 40505, 859-299-3392

Marlane Parra and Debbie Schwebke, Mesilla Park Elementary School, 3101 Bowman Street, Las Cruces, New Mexico, marlane@zianet.com

Joan Peebles, Coordinator, Technology and Learning, Madison Metropolitan School District, 545 West Dayton Street, Room 125, Madison, Wisconsin 53703, 608-663-5228, http://www.madison.k12.wi.us/tnl/tech/techindesx.htm

From Pondering to Learning: Connecting Multiple Intelligences and Service Learning, National Dropout Prevention Center, Clemson University, Corporation for National Service and the National Dropout Prevention Center at Clemson University, used with permission

San Jose Unified School District; Steve Berta, Manager of Student Services and Guidance; Howard Blonsky, Trainer, San Francisco Unified School District; Vicki Butler, Coordinator and Principal for Special Schools, Riverside County Office of Education; Bill Deeb, Director of Research and Evaluation, Alisal Union School District; Marco Orlando, Consultant, California Department of Education; and Andy Stetkevich, Staff Development Specialist, Riverside Unified School District; used with the permission of Howard Blonsky

Success Academy Shadowing Intervention Program: Mike Smith, Principal; Renee Riddle, Shadowing and Intervention Teacher; and Julie Brunner, Guidance Counselor, Pickerington High School, 300 Opportunity Way, Pickerington, OH 43147, julie_brunner@fc.pickerington.k12.oh.us, www. pickerinton.k12.oh.us, 614-833-3038

Leon Swarts, Student, Family, and Community Support Services, Kentucky Department of Education, 500 Metro Street, Frankfort, Kentucky 40601, 502-564-3678

"Team Strategies For Success" by Mary Ann Smialek, © Mary Ann Smialek, published by Scarecrow Press, Inc., 4720 Boston Way, Lanham, Maryland 20706, 800-462-6420

Utah Technology Awareness Project (800) 836-4396, www.uen.org/cgi-bin/websql/utahlink

Index By Strategy

After-School Experiences

Alternative Schooling

Career Education and Workforce Readiness

Community Collaboration

Diverse Learning Styles and Multiple Intelligences

Early Childhood Education

Family Involvement

Individualized Instruction

Instructional Technologies

Mentoring and Tutoring

Professional Development

Reading and Writing Programs

Safe Schools

Service Learning

Systemic Renewal

Index By Grade Level

All Grade Levels

Pre-School

Elementary

Middle/Junior High School

High School